Veterinary Clinical Parasitology

Seventh Edition

Anne M. Zajac

Gary A. Conboy

Under the auspices of the **AAVP**
American Association of Veterinary Parasitologists

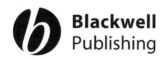 **Blackwell** Publishing

Anne M. Zajac is an associate professor in the Department of Biomedical Sciences and Pathobiology of the Virginia/Maryland Regional College of Veterinary Medicine at Virginia Tech. She received a B.S. in zoology from the University of Michigan and an M.S. in parasitology and D.V.M. from Michigan State University. Dr. Zajac received her Ph.D. in parasitology from Ohio State University.

Gary A. Conboy is an associate professor in the Department of Pathology and Microbiology at the Atlantic Veterinary College, University of Prince Edward Island. He received his B. S. in microbiology and zoology and a D.V.M. and Ph.D. degree from the University of Minnesota.

Blackwell Publishing Professional
2121 State Avenue, Ames, Iowa 50014, USA

Orders: 1-800-862-6657
Office: 1-515-292-0140
Fax: 1-515-292-3348
Web site: www.blackwellprofessional.com

Blackwell Publishing Ltd
9600 Garsington Road, Oxford OX4 2DQ, UK
Tel.: +44 (0)1865 776868

Blackwell Publishing Asia
550 Swanston Street, Carlton, Victoria 3053, Australia
Tel.: +61 (0)3 8359 1011

First, Second editions, 1948, 1955 ©Iowa State College Press
Third, Fourth, Fifth, Sixth editions, 1961, 1970, 1978, 1994 ©Iowa State University Press
Seventh edition, 2006 ©Blackwell Publishing

Library of Congress Cataloging-in-Publication Data

Zajac, Anne M.
    Veterinary clinical parasitology / Anne M. Zajac, Gary A. Conboy.—7th ed.
      p. cm.
    Sixth ed. by Margaret W. Sloss, Russell L. Kemp, and Anne M. Zajac.
    "Under the auspices of the American Association of Veterinary Parasitologists."
    ISBN-13: 978-0-8138-1734-7 (alk. paper)
    ISBN-10: 0-8138-1734-X (alk. paper)
    1. Veterinary clinical parasitology. I. Conboy, Gary A. II. Sloss, Margaret W. (Margaret Wragg), 1901–
Veterinary clinical parasitology. III. American Association of Veterinary Parasitologists. IV. Title.

    SF810.A3S58 2006
    636.089′696—dc22

                                                                                        2005010846

The last digit is the print number: 9 8 7 6 5 4 3 2 1

CONTENTS

PREFACE

Like the 6th edition, the 7th edition of *Veterinary Clinical Parasitology* has been prepared under the auspices of the American Association of Veterinary Parasitologists (AAVP), with contributions of illustrations from many AAVP members. However, the 7th edition is also a departure from the format that has been used in previous editions. Replacing black-and-white illustrations are new color photographs, and brief text material for each parasite has been added to indicate its distribution, life cycle, and importance. We have also expanded the book to include some important parasites not indigenous to North America. What has not changed in this edition of *Veterinary Clinical Parasitology* is the emphasis on morphologic identification of parasites of domestic animals. Although immunologic and molecular techniques are being increasingly applied to the diagnosis of parasitism, veterinary practices worldwide still rely primarily on the humble fecal exam and the other microscopic diagnostic techniques that remain the focus of this edition. These techniques, when done by personnel with the expertise to do them properly, remain an accurate and cost-effective means of diagnosing parasitic infections in animals.

We hope that the changes included in the 7th edition will increase the book's usefulness for veterinarians, veterinary technicians, and others who may be involved in the diagnosis of parasitism in animals.

ACKNOWLEDGMENTS

We are very grateful to the members of the American Association of Veterinary Parasitologists (AAVP) who provided material for this edition of *Veterinary Clinical Parasitology*. Members of AAVP took time from their busy schedules to search through slide collections or even take pictures specifically for this book. Appeals for photographs distributed through the AAVP listserv brought responses from as far away as Germany, Brazil, and Australia. Although the source of each figure is credited in the figure legend (with the exception of photos provided by chapter authors), we would also like to list all the contributors here with our deepest thanks:

Dr. David Baker, School of Veterinary Medicine, Louisiana State University, Baton Rouge, LA
Dr. Byron Blagburn, College of Veterinary Medicine, Auburn University, Auburn, AL
Dr. Dwight Bowman, College of Veterinary Medicine, Cornell University, Ithaca, NY
Dr. George Conder, Pfizer Corporation, Kalamazoo, MI
Dr. Hany Elsheikha and Dr. Charles Mackenzie, College of Veterinary Medicine, Michigan State University, East Lansing, MI
Dr. Bernard Feldman, Virginia-Maryland Regional College of Veterinary Medicine, Virginia Tech, Blacksburg VA
Dr. Alvin Gajadhar, Centre for Animal Parasitology, Canadian Food Inspection Agency, Saskatoon, Saskatchewan, Canada
Dr. Ellis Greiner, College of Veterinary Medicine, University of Florida, Gainesville, FL
Dr. Bruce Hammerberg and Dr. James Flowers, College of Veterinary Medicine, North Carolina State University, Raleigh, NC
Dr. Michael Leib, Virginia-Maryland Regional College of Veterinary Medicine, Virginia Tech, Blacksburg, VA
Dr. David Lindsay, Virginia-Maryland Regional College of Veterinary Medicine, Virginia Tech, Blacksburg, VA
Dr. Gil Myers, Myers Parasitological Service, Magnolia, TN, and Dr. Eugene Lyons, Department of Veterinary Science, University of Kentucky, Lexington KY
Dr. Thomas Nolan, School of Veterinary Medicine, University of Pennsylvania, Philadelphia, PA
Dr. Fernando Paiva, Universidade Federal de Mato Grosso do Sul, Campo Grande, MS, Brazil
Dr. Andrew Peregrine, Ontario Veterinary College, University of Guelph, Guelph, Ontario, Canada
Dr. Steffan Rehbein and Mr. Martin Visser, Merial GmBH, Rohrdorf, Germany
Dr. Craig Reinemeyer, East Tennessee Clinical Research, Knoxville, TN
Dr. Robert Ridley, College of Veterinary Medicine, Kansas State University, Manhattan, KS
Dr. Nick Sangster and Dr. Sally Pope, Faculty of Veterinary Science, University of Sydney, Sydney, New South Wales, Australia
Dr. Philip Scholl, Agricultural Research Service, U.S. Department of Agriculture, University of Nebraska, Lincoln, NE, and Dr. Jerry Weintraub, Agriculture Canada, Lethbridge, Alberta Canada
Dr. Karen Snowden, College of Veterinary Medicine, Texas A&M University, College Station, TX
Dr. T. Bonner Stewart, School of Veterinary Medicine, Louisiana State University, Baton Rouge, LA
Dr. Bert Stromberg and Mr. Gary Averbeck, College of Veterinary Medicine, University of Minnesota, Minneapolis, MN
Dr. Donald B. Thomas, U.S. Department of Agriculture Subtropical Agriculture Research Laboratory, Weslaco, TX
Dr. C.S.F. Williams, Langley, WA

Dr. Jeffrey F. Williams, Vanson HaloSource Inc., Redmond, WA

Dr. Tom Yazwinski and Mr. Chris Tucker, Department of Animal Science, University of Arkansas, Fayetteville, AK

Dr. Gary Zimmerman, Zimmerman Research, West Montana, Livingston, MT

AUTHORS

Anne M. Zajac, DVM, PhD
Department of Biomedical Sciences and Pathobiology
Virginia-Maryland Regional College of Veterinary Medicine
Virginia Tech
Blacksburg, VA 24061

Gary A. Conboy, DVM, PhD
Department of Pathobiology and Microbiology
Atlantic Veterinary College
University of Prince Edward Island
Charlottetown, Prince Edward Island C1A 4P3
Canada

Ellis C. Greiner, PhD
Department of Infectious Diseases
College of Veterinary Medicine
University of Florida
Box J-137
Gainesville, FL 32610

Stephen A. Smith, DVM, PhD
Department of Biomedical Sciences and Pathobiology
Virginia-Maryland Regional College of Veterinary Medicine
Virginia Tech
Blacksburg, VA 24061

Veterinary Clinical Parasitology

Seventh Edition

Fecal Examination for the Diagnosis of Parasitism

The fecal examination for diagnosis of parasitic infections is probably the most common laboratory procedure performed in veterinary practice. Fecal examination can reveal the presence of parasites in several body systems. Parasites inhabiting the digestive system produce eggs, larvae, or cysts that leave the body of the host by way of the feces. Occasionally, even adult helminth parasites may be seen in feces, especially when the host has enteritis. Parasitic worm eggs or larvae from the respiratory system are usually coughed into the pharynx and swallowed, and they too appear in feces. Mange or scab mites may be licked or nibbled from the skin, thus accounting for their appearance in the feces. Many parasitic forms seen in feces have characteristic morphologic features that, when combined with knowledge of the host, are diagnostic for a particular species of parasite. On the other hand, certain parasites produce similar eggs, oocysts, etc. and cannot be identified to the species level (e.g., many of the strongylid-type eggs from livestock). Fecal examination may also reveal to a limited extent the status of digestion, as shown by the presence of undigested muscle, starch, or fat droplets.

COLLECTION OF FECAL SAMPLES

Fecal exams should be conducted on fresh fecal material. If fecal samples are submitted to the laboratory after being in the environment for hours or days, fragile protozoan trophozoites will have died and disappeared. The eggs of some nematodes can hatch within a few days in warm weather, and identification of nematode larvae is far more difficult than recognizing the familiar eggs of common species. Also, free-living nematodes rapidly invade a fecal sample on the ground, and differentiation of hatched parasite larvae from these free-living species can be time-consuming and difficult.

Owners of small animals should be instructed to collect at least several grams of feces immediately after observing defecation. This will ensure the proper identification of the sample with the client's pet (i.e., a sample from a stray animal will not be collected) and that feces rather than vomitus or other material is collected. The limited amount of feces recovered from the rectum on a thermometer or fecal loop should not be relied on for routine parasitologic examination, since many infections that produce only small numbers of eggs will be missed. Owners should be instructed to store fecal samples in the refrigerator if the sample will not be submitted for examination for more than an hour or two after collection.

Feces should be collected directly from the rectum of large animals. This is particularly important if the sample is to be examined for lungworm larvae, since contaminating free-living nematodes and hatched first-stage larvae of gastrointestinal nematodes may be confused with lungworm larvae. If rectal samples are unavailable, owners should be asked to collect feces immediately after observing defecation. The process of development and hatching of common strongylid eggs can be slowed by refrigeration. Development is also reduced when air is excluded from the sample by placing the collected feces in a plastic bag and pressing out the air before sealing the bag.

STORAGE AND SHIPMENT OF FECAL SAMPLES

If collected feces cannot be examined within a few hours, the sample should be refrigerated until it can be tested. Feces should not be frozen, because freezing can distort parasite eggs. If a sample needs to be evaluated for the presence of protozoan trophozoites like *Giardia* and trichomonads, it should be examined within 30 minutes after collection. The trophozoite is the active, feeding form of the parasite and is not adapted to environmental survival; it dies soon after being passed in the feces.

If fresh fecal material is submitted to another laboratory for examination, it should be packaged with cold packs. Helminth eggs may also be preserved with an equal volume of 5–10% buffered formalin. The use of formalin for fixation of samples has the additional benefit of inactivating many other infectious organisms that may be present. Special fixatives, such as polyvinyl alcohol (PVA), are required to preserve protozoan trophozoites and are not routinely used in veterinary practices.

Slides prepared from flotation tests do not travel well, even if the coverslip is ringed with nail polish, since hyperosmotic flotation solutions will usually make parasite eggs or larvae unrecognizable within hours of preparing the slide. However, slides from flotation tests can be preserved for several hours to several days by placing them in a refrigerator in a covered container containing moist paper towels to maintain high humidity. It is best to place applicator sticks under the slide to prevent it from becoming too wet.

FECAL EXAM PROCEDURES

Before performing specific tests on the fecal sample, its general appearance should be noted; consistency, color, and the presence of blood or mucus may all be indicative of specific parasitic infections. Hookworm disease in dogs, for example, commonly produces dark, tarry feces, whereas diarrheic feces caused by whipworms may contain excess mucus and frank blood. The presence of adult parasites or tapeworm segments should also be noted.

Fecal Flotation

The technique most commonly used in veterinary medicine for examination of feces is the fecal flotation test. This procedure concentrates parasite eggs and cysts and removes debris. Fecal flotation is based on the principle that parasite material present in the feces is less dense than the fluid flotation medium and thus will float to the top of the container, where it can be collected for microscopic evaluation. Flotation tests are easy and inexpensive to perform, but in busy practices the choice of flotation solution and test procedure often does not receive much consideration, despite the substantial effect these choices can have on the sensitivity of flotation exams.

Choice and Preparation of Flotation Solutions

Many different substances can be used to make flotation solutions. The higher the specific gravity (SpG) of the flotation solution, the greater the variety of parasite eggs that will float. However, as the SpG increases, more debris will also float and the risk of damage to eggs from the hyperosmotic solution also increases. These factors limit the range of useful flotation solutions to SpG ranging from approximately 1.18 to 1.3. The flotation solutions widely used in veterinary parasitology include sugar solution and various salt solutions.

Probably the most commonly used flotation solution in the USA is a commercially available sodium nitrate solution (Fecasol®, Evsco Pharmaceuticals, Buena, NJ 08310), with SpG 1.2. This solution is readily available and will float common helminth eggs and protozoan cysts. However, *Giardia* cysts are rapidly distorted and difficult to identify in sodium nitrate flotations. Because of the importance of *Giardia* in small-animal practice, a more useful flotation solution is a 33% zinc sulfate solution (SpG 1.18). This solution does not cause such rapid destruction of *Giardia* cysts and allows them to be more easily recognized in flotation preparations. Zinc sulfate solution can be made in veterinary practices or purchased commercially. Neither of these flotation solutions will float most trematode eggs and some tapeworm and very dense nematode eggs.

Saturated solutions of sodium chloride (SpG 1.20) and of magnesium sulfate (Epsom salts, SpG 1.32) can also be prepared for use in flotation procedures. Saturated sodium nitrate solution can also be used and will have a higher specific gravity (1.33) than the commercially available product. The saturated solutions have the advantages of being inexpensive, easy to purchase or prepare, and effective in floating common parasite eggs. However, like sodium nitrate and zinc sulfate, they will not float very dense helminth eggs (most trematode eggs, some tapeworm and nematode eggs). These solutions also quickly distort *Giardia* cysts. Another common solution used in routine flotation exams is Sheather's sugar solution (SpG 1.2–1.25). Sheather's solution is recommended for recovery of *Cryptosporidium* in fecal samples and may be more effective than some salt solutions for recovery of equine tapeworm eggs. Sheather's sugar solution does not appear to be as effective as 33% $ZnSO_4$ solution for detection of *Giardia* (see Zajac, Johnson, and King 2002). Sheather's solution is inexpensive and easy to prepare, but it is sticky and rather messy to use in a laboratory area. The advantages and disadvantages of these solutions are shown in Table 1.1 and instructions for preparing them are given below.

Although the SpG of flotation solutions is not often measured in practices, it can be easily de-

Table 1.1. Comparison of commonly used flotation solutions

Flotation Solution	Specific Gravity	Advantages	Disadvantages
Sodium nitrate (NaNO₃) Fecasol® (Saturated NaNO₃)	1.2 1.33	Floats common helminth and protozoa eggs and cysts.	Distorts *Giardia* cysts rapidly. Does not float most flukes and some unusual tapeworm and nematode eggs.
33% Zinc sulfate (ZnSO₄)	1.18	Floats common helminth and protozoa eggs and cysts. Preferred for *Giardia* and some lungworm larvae.	Does not float most flukes and some unusual tapeworm and nematode eggs.
Saturated sodium chloride (NaCl)	1.2	Floats common helminth and protozoa eggs and cysts.	Distorts *Giardia* cysts rapidly. Does not float most flukes and some unusual tapeworm and nematode eggs.
Saturated magnesium sulfate (Epsom salts)	1.32	Floats common helminth and protozoa eggs and cysts.	Distorts *Giardia* cysts rapidly. Does not float most flukes and some unusual tapeworm and nematode eggs.
Sheather's sugar solution	1.25	Floats common helminth and protozoa eggs and cysts. Preferred for *Cryptosporidium* oocysts.	Does not float most flukes and some unusual tapeworm and nematode eggs. Less sensitive than ZnSO₄ for *Giardia*. Creates sticky surfaces.

termined with an inexpensive hydrometer from a scientific supply company. A hydrometer will last indefinitely and should be considered part of quality control for the veterinary practice laboratory.

33% ZINC SULFATE SOLUTION (SPG 1.18)

1. Combine 330 g zinc sulfate with water to reach a volume of 1000 ml.
2. Additional water or zinc sulfate can be added to produce a SpG of 1.18 (if zinc sulfate solution is used with formalinized feces, the SpG should be increased to 1.20).
3. Check the SpG with a hydrometer.

SATURATED SODIUM CHLORIDE (NACL, SPG 1.2) OR MAGNESIUM SULFATE SOLUTION (MGSO₄, SPG 1.32)

1. Add salt to warm tap water until no more salt goes into solution and the excess settles on the bottom of the container.
2. To ensure that the solution is fully saturated, it should be allowed to stand overnight at room temperature. If remaining salt crystals dissolve overnight, more can be added to ensure that the solution is saturated.
3. Check the SpG with a hydrometer, recognizing that the SpG of saturated solutions will vary slightly with environmental temperature.

SHEATHER'S SUGAR SOLUTION (SPG 1.2–1.25)

1. Combine 355 ml (12 fluid ounces of water) and 454 g (1 pound) of granulated sugar (sucrose). Corn syrup and dextrose are not suitable substitutes.
2. Dissolve the sugar in the water by stirring over low or indirect heat (e.g., the top half of a double boiler). If the container is placed on a high direct heat source, the sugar may caramelize instead of dissolving in the water.
3. After the sugar is dissolved and the solution has cooled to room temperature, add 6 ml formaldehyde USP to prevent microbial growth (30 ml of 10% formalin can also be used, with the volume of water reduced to 330 ml).
4. Check the SpG with a hydrometer.

Flotation Procedures

No matter how the flotation procedure is performed, the principle is the same. After mixing the flotation solution and the fecal sample together, the less dense material eventually floats to the top. This process can occur either by letting the mixture sit on the benchtop for a specified time or by centrifuging the mixture. Regardless of the flotation solution used, centrifugation makes the flotation occur more rapidly and efficiently. Many practitioners like to use convenient commercial flotation kits that provide a container for collection of the sample and performing the test. However, the convenience of the kits is offset by the loss of sensitivity in the fecal exam procedure. A smaller amount of feces is used and the test cannot be centrifuged.

The increased sensitivity of the centrifugation procedure is particularly important in infections where the diagnostic form of the parasite is present in low numbers (e.g., *Trichuris* and *Giardia* infections in dogs and cats). Centrifugation is also necessary when using 33% $ZnSO_4$ or sugar solution because of the slightly lower SpG of $ZnSO_4$ solution and the high viscosity of sugar solution, both of which retard the flotation process. Many veterinary practices do not centrifuge their flotation tests and rely on the traditional benchtop incubation technique, thereby reducing the sensitivity of their fecal exams.

CENTRIFUGAL FECAL FLOTATION PROCEDURE

This procedure should be used with Sheather's sugar and 33% $ZnSO_4$ flotation solutions and is also recommended for other flotation procedures.

1. Mix 3–5 g (about 1 teaspoonful) of feces with a small amount of flotation solution in a paper or plastic cup. Cat feces and small ruminant pellets, which are sometimes too hard to break up easily, can be ground with a mortar and pestle or allowed to soak in water until they become softer.

   If the sample appears to contain a large amount of fat or mucus, an initial water wash is performed and water should be used in Step 1. The water wash can be eliminated for most fecal samples of normal appearance.
2. Strain the mixture of feces and flotation solution (or feces and water if a water wash is performed) through a double layer of cheesecloth or gauze. A tea strainer can also be used.
3. Pour the mixture into a 15 ml centrifuge tube. If the rotor on the centrifuge is not angled (i.e., if the tubes hang straight when not spinning), the centrifuge tube can be filled with flotation solution until a reverse meniscus is formed and a coverslip added (Fig. 1.1). The tube is spun with the coverslip. The centrifugal force generated by the centrifuge will hold the coverslip in place. If the centrifuge has an angled rotor, fill the tube as full as possible and place in the centrifuge.
4. Spin the mixture in a benchtop centrifuge for about 5 minutes at approximately 500–650 G (650 G is 2500 rpm on a 4-inch rotor), regardless of whether the feces have been mixed with water or with the flotation solution. If a specific G force and speed setting cannot be determined, spinning the tube at the same speed used to separate serum from blood cells is sufficient.

   If the initial spin is a water wash, the supernatant should be discarded, the sediment resuspended with flotation solution, and Steps 3 and 4 repeated.
5. Allow the centrifuge to stop without using the brake. The slight jerking that results from use of the brake may dislodge parasites from the surface layer.
6. Following centrifugation, there are several ways to harvest the surface layer of fluid containing parasite eggs. If the tube has been spun with the coverslip in place, lift the coverslip off the tube and quickly place it on a microscope slide. When the tube is spun without the coverslip, remove the tube from the centrifuge after spinning and place in a test tube rack. Fill the tube with additional flotation solution to form a reverse meniscus. Place a coverslip on the tube and allow it to sit for an additional 5–10 minutes before removing the coverslip and placing it on a slide.

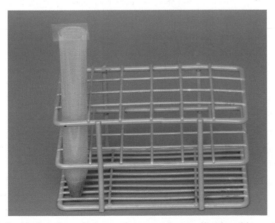

Fig. 1.1. Centrifuge tube filled with flotation solution to the top and coverslip placed in contact with the fluid column.

Alternatively, after the centrifuge comes to a stop, gently touch the surface of the fluid in the tube with a glass rod, microbiological loop, or base of a small glass tube and then quickly touch the rod to a microscope slide to transfer the drop or two of adhering fluid. This procedure will be less efficient than allowing the tube to stand with a coverslip in place.

BENCHTOP (SIMPLE) FLOTATION PROCEDURE

When a centrifugal flotation procedure cannot be performed, sodium nitrate and saturated salt solutions can be used in a benchtop flotation test, although the sensitivity of the test will be reduced. This technique is not recommended for 33% $ZnSO_4$ or sugar flotation tests.

1. Mix several grams (a teaspoonful) of feces with the flotation solution in a cup.
2. Strain the mixture through cheesecloth or a tea strainer.
3. Pour into a test tube, pill vial, or container provided in a commercial kit. Add enough mixture or additional flotation fluid until there is a reverse meniscus on the top of the container. Place a coverslip on the fluid drop at the top.
4. Allow the flotation to stand for at least 10 minutes, remove the coverslip, place it on a slide, and examine. If the test is allowed to stand for too long, the salt may crystallize on the edges of the coverslip so that it will not lie flat on the slide.

FLOTATION SLIDES

Fecal flotation slides should be scanned using the 10× objective lens of the microscope (since most microscopes also have an eyepiece magnification of 10×, using the 10× objective gives a total magnification of 100×). Although most helminth eggs can be detected with the 4× objective, protozoan parasites are easily missed and this low power should not be used for scanning. The 40× lens should be used when there is uncertainty about the identity of structures on the slide and for scanning slides for *Cryptosporidium* oocysts. In some practices, to save expense coverslips are not used. However, slides without coverslips dry out faster, do not have a flat plane of focus, and cannot be examined with the 40× lens, with the result that some parasites will be identified incorrectly or missed entirely.

EGG-COUNTING PROCEDURES (QUANTITATIVE FECAL EXAMS)

Egg-counting techniques are also flotation tests and are recommended primarily to estimate the extent of parasite egg contamination on pastures grazed by infected animals or to determine the efficacy of drug treatment (discussed in a later section in this chapter). Egg counts are of limited value in making judgments about the clinical condition of individual animals because many factors affect egg production, including parasite species, individual host immunity, and stage of infection. Also, counts performed on combined samples from a number of animals may not accurately reflect parasitism within that herd.

The easiest quantitative test to perform is the Modified McMaster Test. This test requires the use of special reusable slides, which can be purchased inexpensively from several suppliers (Fig. 1.2; suppliers of McMaster slides include Chalex Corporation, 5004 228th Avenue SE, Issaquah, WA 98029 USA [www.vetslides.com]; Focal Point, P.O. Box 12832, Onderstepoort 0110, South Africa [www.mcmaster.co.za]; and JA Whitlock & Co., PO Box 51, Eastwood, NSW 2122, Australia [www.whitlock.com.au]). Any of the saturated salt solutions can be used in this technique. The Modified McMaster Test has a sensitivity of 25 or 50 eggs per gram of feces depending on the amount of materials used. This level of sensitivity is acceptable in most situations since parasite control programs do not usually require detection of lower egg numbers. However, if egg counts of

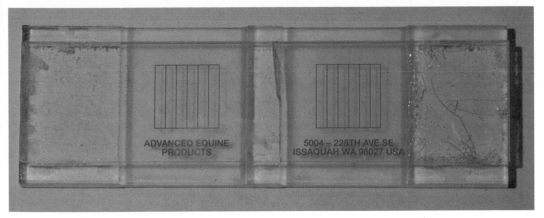

Fig. 1.2. McMaster slide used in the Modified McMaster procedure for quantitative egg counts.

less than 50 are expected (e.g., in adult cattle) or it is important to detect very low numbers of eggs, the Wisconsin Sugar Flotation Test can be used. This procedure permits detection of less than 1 egg/g of fecal material but is more time-consuming to perform.

Regardless of the procedure used to count parasites, the most important element is consistency. Each step of the procedure should be performed in the same way for every sample.

Modified McMaster Test

1. Combine 4 g of fecal material with 56 ml of flotation solution to yield a total volume of 60 ml. The test can also be performed with 2 g of feces and 28 ml of flotation solution when only small amounts of feces are available. A digital kitchen scale that weighs in 1 g increments can be used to measure feces.
2. Mix well and strain through cheesecloth if desired. The mixture does not have to be strained, but it will be much easier to read the slide if large pieces of debris are removed.
3. Immediately fill each chamber of the McMaster slide with the mixture using a Pasteur pipette or syringe. The entire chamber must be filled, not just the area under the grid. If large air bubbles are present, remove the fluid and refill.
4. Allow the slide to sit for at least 5 minutes before examining to allow the flotation process to occur.
5. Look at the slide with the 10× lens, focusing on the top layer, which contains the air bubbles. At this level, the lines of the grid will also be in focus. Count eggs, oocysts, etc. in each lane of both chambers. Each type of parasite should be counted separately. In some cases, eggs can be identified to genus or perhaps to species (e.g., *Strongyloides, Trichuris,* and *Nematodirus*), whereas others must be counted as a category of parasites (coccidia, strongylid eggs).

To determine the number of parasite eggs per gram of feces, add the counts for both chambers for each parasite. Most commercial McMaster slides are calibrated so that the grid in each chamber allows you to count the eggs present in 0.15 ml of fecal mixture. If you add the results of both chambers, you have counted the eggs present in 0.3 ml, which is 1/200th of the total volume of 60 ml; therefore, the number of eggs must be multiplied by 200. However, since you began with 4 g of feces, the result must be divided by 4 to yield eggs per gram of feces. Multiplying by 200 and dividing by 4 is equivalent to multiplying the number of eggs counted by 50. Therefore, seeing 1 egg is equivalent to 50 eggs/g. The same level of sensitivity can be achieved by using 2 g of fecal material and 28 ml of flotation solution. The smaller amount of feces may be preferred when evaluating small lambs or kids. If a sensitivity of 25 eggs/g is desired, the McMaster test should be performed with 4 g of feces and 26 ml of flotation solution (results are then multiplied by 100 and divided by 4 as described above).

Wisconsin Egg-Counting Technique

The Wisconsin Egg-Counting Test is essentially a Sheather's sugar flotation procedure performed with specific quantities of feces and flotation fluid.

1. Combine 5 g of feces and 15 ml of water in a cup. A digital kitchen scale is a convenient way to measure fecal samples.
2. Mix thoroughly and strain through cheesecloth or a tea strainer into a 15 ml centrifuge tube.
3. Centrifuge the tube as described above in the procedure for the centrifugal flotation technique.
4. After spinning, discard supernatant and resuspend the pellet in Sheather's sugar solution.

   If desired, the initial water wash can be omitted and the sample mixed initially with flotation solution. Alternatively, in the Modified Wisconsin procedure, 22 ml of flotation solution is mixed with 5 g of feces, and the resulting mixture is divided between two tubes. This modification increases the accuracy of the procedure.
5. Either spin the tube with a coverslip in place or allow additional incubation after spinning as described for the centrifugal flotation procedure.
6. Remove the coverslip and examine with the 10× objective lens, systematically scanning the slide and counting eggs or cysts of each parasite species or group separately. Care must be taken to ensure that each microscope field on the coverslip is examined once but only once so that no eggs are missed or counted twice.

   This technique allows quantification of at least 1 egg/5 g of feces.

Additional Procedures for Fecal Examination

The following procedures are used for identification of specific parasitic infections.

Direct Smear and Stained Fecal Smears

The direct smear is used to identify protozoan trophozoites (*Giardia*, trichomonads, amoebae, etc.) or other structures that float poorly or are readily distorted by flotation solutions. Because very little feces is used, the sensitivity of this test is low. It is not recommended for routine fecal examinations.

1. Mix a very small amount of feces with a drop of saline on a microscope slide to produce a layer through which newsprint can be read. Saline should be used because water will destroy protozoan trophozoites.
2. Use a coverslip to push large particles of debris to the side and place the coverslip on the slide. Examine with 10× and 40× magnification. The 100× lens (oil immersion) cannot be used effectively with fecal smears.
3. If the fecal layer is too thick, it will be impossible to see small, colorless protozoa moving in the field. Movement is the principal characteristic that allows recognition of trophozoites in fresh fecal smears. A drop of Lugol's iodine will enhance the internal structures of protozoan cysts but will also kill trophozoites present. To maximize the use of this test, it is best to look at an unstained smear before adding iodine.

Fecal smears can also be stained for identification of intestinal protozoa. Several stains can be used for identification of *Cryptosporidium*, including Ziehl-Neelsen, Kinyoun, carbol-fuchsin, and Giemsa stains. Trichrome stain is widely used in human medicine for detection of *Giardia* cysts. In general, however, stains are not used extensively in veterinary practices and are not required for the identification of parasitic organisms. For details on performing these stains, a standard text on human parasitologic diagnosis should be consulted.

Fecal Sedimentation

A sedimentation procedure is used to isolate eggs of flukes and some other tapeworms and nematodes whose eggs do not float readily in common flotation solutions. In the simple sedimentation test, tap water is combined with feces and allowed to settle briefly before the supernatant is removed. This allows removal of fine particulate material, but unlike the flotation exam, sedimentation tests have only limited concentrating ability. Fat and mucus can be removed from the fecal sample if a centrifugal sedimentation exam is performed using ethyl acetate. Unfortunately, ethyl acetate is toxic and very flammable. It should be stored in a flameproof cabinet and used only in well-ventilated areas. An alternative to ethyl acetate is Hemo-De, available through Fischer Scientific (www.fischerscientific.com), which is generally regarded as a safe compound and appears to give equivalent results in a centrifugal sedimentation procedure (see Neimester et al. 1987).

The Flukefinder® is a commercially available apparatus for performing sedimentation tests in the laboratory. It utilizes several screens to rapidly remove fecal debris. This device is very useful in practices conducting routine fecal examinations for flukes. The Flukefinder and instructions for its use can be obtained from Visual Differences, 5051C Old Pullman Road, Moscow, ID 83842 USA.

SIMPLE SEDIMENTATION TEST

1. Mix about 100 ml of water with about 10 g of feces and place in a beaker or other container.
2. Allow mixture to sit for 1 hour and then decant the supernatant.
3. Add more water, mix, and repeat the sedimentation procedure.
4. Stir remaining mixture and place a few drops on a microscope slide. If desired, add 1 drop of 0.1% methylene blue. The methylene blue will stain the background debris blue but will not stain fluke eggs, which will stand out with a yellowish brown color.
5. Coverslip and scan the slide at the 10× magnification.

A smaller amount of feces and water can be used, placed in a test tube, and left to sit for 3–5 minutes between decantation steps. Addition of a drop of dishwashing soap to the water used in the test helps to free eggs from surrounding debris.

CENTRIFUGAL SEDIMENTATION TEST

1. Mix 1 g of feces with about 10 ml of 10% buffered formalin or water. Pour mixture into a 15 ml centrifuge tube (with cap) until it is one-half to three-quarters full.
2. Add ethyl acetate (see above discussion of safety) or Hemo-De until the tube is almost full. Because organic solvents may dissolve some plastic centrifuge tubes, it is recommended that glass or polypropylene tubes be used for performing this test.
3. Cap and shake the tube approximately 50 times.
4. Centrifuge for 3–5 minutes at about 500 G (as for centrifugal flotation procedure).
5. When the tube is removed from the centrifuge, it will have three layers: (*a*) an upper layer containing ethyl acetate, fat, and debris; (*b*) a middle layer containing formalin or water and fine particulate matter; and (*c*) a bottom layer of sediment. Using an applicator stick, loosen the top

debris plug that sticks to the sides of the tube, then decant the supernatant leaving only the bottom sediment.

6. Resuspend the sediment in a few drops of water or formalin, place 1 or 2 drops of the sediment on a slide, coverslip, and examine with the 10× microscope objective.

Baermann Test

The Baermann Test is used to isolate larvae from fecal samples and is employed most often to diagnose lungworm infections. *It is very important that the fecal sample be fresh.* If feces of a grazing animal are being examined and an old sample is used, strongylid or *Strongyloides* eggs may have hatched, or free-living nematodes may have invaded the sample, making nematode identification much more difficult. In small-animal samples, hookworm eggs may hatch very quickly and can be confused with lungworm or *Strongyloides* larvae.

A Baermann Test requires equipment to hold the fecal sample in water so that larvae can migrate out and be collected. This can now be most easily accomplished with the use of a plastic wine glass with a hollow stem. In the absence of disposable wine glasses, the original Baermann apparatus can be used. This consists of a funnel clamped to a metal stand. A short piece of tubing with a clamp is attached to the end of the funnel. Larvae in feces placed either in the bowl of the wine glass or in the funnel migrate out of the sample and fall down into the hollow stem or the tubing above the clamp, where they can be easily collected (Fig. 1.3).

1. Place at least 10 g of feces in a piece of double-layer cheesecloth. Gather the cheesecloth around the sample so that it is fully enclosed. Use a rubber band to fasten the cheesecloth, and pass through the rubber band two applicator sticks (pencils, etc.), which will rest on the edges of the glass or funnel and suspend the sample. Alternatively, place the sample on a suspended piece of wire mesh or sieve.
2. Fill the funnel or wine glass with lukewarm water. Make sure that the corners of the cheesecloth do not hang over the edge of the funnel or glass, because they will act as wicks for the water.
3. Allow the sample to sit for at least 8 hours, preferably overnight.

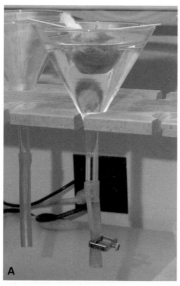
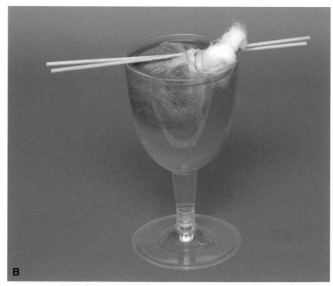

Fig. 1.3. On the left is the traditional Baermann apparatus consisting of a suspended funnel with clamped tubing attached. For diagnostic testing of fecal samples it is much more convenient to perform the Baermann exam with a disposable plastic wine glass (*right*).

4. If using the disposable plastic glass, remove the fecal sample and collect the material at the bottom of the hollow stem using a Pasteur pipette or syringe. Transfer some of the fluid to a microscope slide, coverslip, and examine with the 4× or 10× objective lens.
5. If using the funnel, release the clamp and collect the first 10 ml of fluid into a centrifuge tube. Spin as for a flotation exam, discard the supernatant, and examine the sediment. Alternatively, the very steady-handed can carefully loosen the clamp and collect the first 3 or 4 drops onto a microscope slide.

Immunological Methods

Immunological methods have been important in the diagnosis of blood and tissue parasites for many years, and they are now being used increasingly for identification of specific parasites in fecal samples. Although these techniques cannot currently replace morphologic exam of feces as a routine screening procedure for multiple infections, they are useful for specific diagnosis of some protozoan parasites that are detected in feces. Currently, commercial indirect fluorescent antibody (IFA) and enzyme immunosorbent assays (EIA) kits are available for diagnosis of *Cryptosporidium* and *Giardia*. These tests detect the parasite or parasite antigens in the feces; they are not host species specific. The IFA and EIA techniques are more widely used in parasitic diagnosis using blood samples and are further discussed in Chapter 3.

QUALITY CONTROL FOR FECAL EXAM PROCEDURES

Although the concept of quality control is not often applied to fecal exams, attention to both equipment and training will help ensure that fecal exams are consistently done correctly.

1. Keep microscopes in good repair. Objective lenses and eyepieces should be routinely cleaned with lens cleaner and lens paper. Have microscopes professionally cleaned and checked every few years.
2. Check the specific gravity of flotation solutions with a hydrometer to ensure that they will recover parasites effectively.
3. Use an ocular micrometer (see section on microscope calibration later in this chapter) to measure structures seen on fecal exams. If possible, recalibrate the microscope when it is cleaned.
4. Make sure that personnel performing the fecal exams are adequately trained. It is not unusual for untrained assistants to be given rudimentary instruction on performing flotation tests and then be assigned to do them. Under these circumstances it is hardly surprising that air bubbles are identified as coccidia and that smaller parasites are missed entirely.
5. As a check on the diagnostic accuracy of in-clinic fecal exams, periodically submit duplicate portions of fecal samples to a diagnostic laboratory. Both negative and positive samples should be submitted.

USE OF THE MICROSCOPE

There are several points to remember in using the microscope to examine preparations for parasites.

1. Use the 10× objective lens of the microscope for scanning slides. This will provide a total magnification of 100× since most microscope eyepieces contain an additional 10× lens. Start in one corner and systematically scan the entire slide. The 40× objective lens (400× total magnification with eyepiece) is useful for closer examination or for looking for very small organisms

such as *Giardia* or *Cryptosporidium*. The 100× (oil immersion) lens should not be used for flotation preparations. Not only is it likely that flotation solution will contact the lens and possibly damage it, but the pressure of the lens on the coverslip will create currents in the fluid on the slide, keeping everything in motion and making examination of structures difficult.

2. Most parasite eggs and larvae have little or no color and do not stand out well, so it is important to maximize the contrast between the parasites and their backgrounds. Using a microscope with a substage condenser kept in the low position while scanning slides is the best way to increase contrast. Even when a substage condenser is not available, reducing the intensity of light projected on the slide is generally advisable, either by decreasing the microscope rheostat setting or by reducing the aperture of the iris diaphragm. A higher power used for close examination will, of course, require an increased amount of light.

3. When reading a slide, it is helpful to focus up and down with the fine focus to change somewhat the plane of focus. Frequently, worm eggs will be at a slightly different level than protozoan cysts or oocysts, and a small manipulation of the fine focus may make structures more readily visible (Figs. 1.4–1.6).

Microscope Calibration

The ability to measure the size of parasite eggs, oocysts, etc. is very helpful when identifying unusual parasites or where different organisms are similar in appearance but differ in size. For measurements, a micrometer disc (Fig. 1.7) is inserted into the ocular tube of the microscope and calibrated against a known reference in the form of a stage micrometer (Fig. 1.8). Each objective lens of the microscope must be individually calibrated with the ocular lens/micrometer combination to be used, and the calibrations should be posted close to the microscope for easy reference. The calibration will be accurate only for that particular microscope ocular and objective combination. Even if each lens is not calibrated with the stage micrometer, the ocular grid will provide a consistent reference against which to compare objects seen in fecal samples. These ocular micrometer discs and stage micrometers are not expensive and can be purchased from scientific catalogues that include microscope equipment.

Calibration of the 40× objective illustrates the procedure for calibration of the micrometer.

1. To calibrate the 40× objective, place the stage micrometer on the stage of the microscope and focus until the lines are sharp. In the example (Fig. 1.9), the stage micrometer is 1 mm (1000 µm) long and is divided into 100 parts; thus each small division of the stage micrometer represents 10 µm.

2. Superimpose any convenient numbered line of the ocular micrometer (usually the 0 mark) on a convenient line of the stage micrometer (the first large line in the example). The field should now resemble Figure 1.9.

3. Find the two lines that are exactly superimposed. In the example, line 49 of the ocular micrometer falls exactly on line 11 of the stage micrometer. Thus 49 divisions of the unknown ocular micrometer represent 11 divisions, each 10 µm in length, for a total of 110 µm. To complete the calibration, divide 110 µm by 49 divisions, resulting in a calibration factor of 2.24 µm per division for the ocular micrometer in the example.

4. Repeat this procedure for each objective lens to be calibrated on the microscope.

To use the calibrated microscope, superimpose the ocular micrometer scale on an egg or cyst and count the number of divisions subtended by the specimen, for example, 12. Multiply 12 by the calibration factor (2.24 for the 400 lens in the example; $12 \times 2.24 = 26.88$ µm, the size of the object measured).

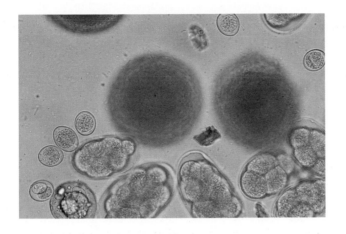

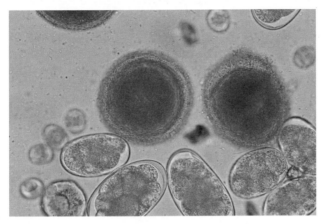

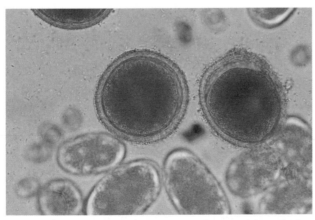

Figures 1.4–1.6. The importance of small changes in the microscope focus can be seen in these three photos of the same field in a canine fecal flotation test. In each case, a slight manipulation of the fine focus brings a different parasite into clearer view (first *Isospora* oocysts, then hookworm eggs, and finally *Toxocara* eggs) since each egg or oocyst type may be present on a slightly different level.

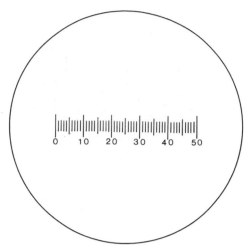

Fig. 1.7. A typical ocular micrometer of 50 divisions. The divisions have no meaning until calibrated against a stage micrometer.

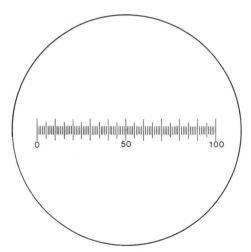

Fig. 1.8. A typical stage micrometer of 1 mm total length. Each division represents 10 μm.

PSEUDOPARASITES AND SPURIOUS PARASITES

Fecal samples may contain deceptive "pseudoparasites" and "spurious parasites." Pseudoparasites are ingested objects that resemble parasite forms; these include pollen grains, plant hairs, grain mites, mold spores, and a variety of harmless plant and animal debris (Figs. 1.10–1.13). "Spurious parasites" are parasite eggs or cysts from one species of host that may be found in the feces of a scavenger or predator host as the result of coprophagy or predation (Figs. 1.14–1.15). One of the best ways to avoid misidentifying these pseudo- and spurious parasites is to appreciate the variety of parasites that normally infect a host species. If a fecal sample contains a possible pseudoparasite or spurious parasite, it is best to repeat the examination with another sample collected at a later time.

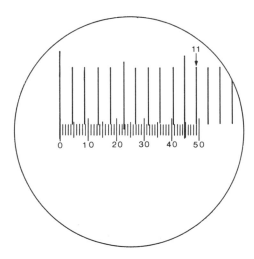

Fig. 1.9. Appearance at 40× of an ocular micrometer being calibrated with a 10 μm/division stage micrometer. Note the conjunction of line 11 of the stage micrometer with line 49 of the ocular micrometer.

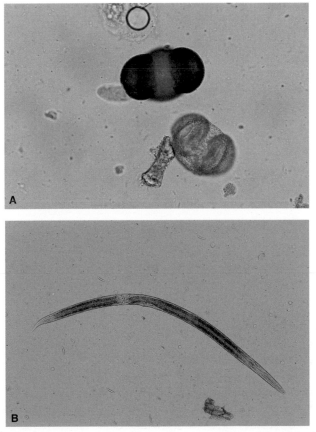

Fig. 1.10A and B. Examples of pseudoparasites. (*A*) Pine pollen is a common pseudoparasite found in fecal samples of many animals (40×). (*B*) Adult free-living nematodes are also commonly found in fecal samples collected from the ground. These nematodes can rapidly invade fecal material. The presence of adults and variation in size and morphology (indicating different stages of the life cycle) are helpful in distinguishing these worms from parasitic larvae.

TECHNIQUES FOR EVALUATION OF STRONGYLID NEMATODES IN GRAZING ANIMALS

Grazing animals are infected with a variety of species of strongylid nematodes whose eggs are not easily differentiated. In veterinary practices, it is usually unnecessary to identify individual species because treatment and control are generally directed to the entire group of nematodes rather than to a single species. If specific identification of the strongylids present in an animal or group of animals is needed, the most convenient method for identification is culture of eggs to the third larval stage. In ruminants, these larvae can then be identified to parasite genus. In horses, this technique can be used to identify large and small strongyle larvae and identify some genera specifically.

Fecal Culture

1. Fresh feces from cattle or horses should be thoroughly mixed and moistened with water if dry. Feces should not be wet, only moist. Larvae do not survive well in very wet fecal material. If cattle feces are liquid, peat moss or vermiculite can be added to create a more suitable consistency. Sheep and goat pellets can be cultured as they are, without breaking them up. Rectal fecal samples are preferred for culture to prevent contamination with free-living nematodes.
2. Place feces in a cup or jar in a layer several centimeters deep. The container should have a loose cover to deter flies. The culture can be kept at room temperature for 10–20 days or at 27°C for 7 days. Daily stirring of the culture will inhibit mold growth and circulate oxygen for the developing larvae. Additional water can be added if feces begin to dry out.
3. Following the culture period, harvest larvae with the Baermann Test described above.

Larva Identification

To identify larvae, place a drop or two of liquid containing larvae from the Baermann procedure on a microscope slide. Add an equal amount of Lugol's iodine. The iodine will kill and stain the larvae so that they can be examined closely.

Larvae recovered from ruminant fecal material can be most easily identified by a combina-tion of size and shape. The shape of the head and tip of the tail and the length of the sheath extending beyond the tail at the posterior end of the larva are important characteristics (Figs. 1.16–1.17 and Table 1.2).

Horses are infected with over 30 species of strongylid parasites, but only a few can be identified on the basis of the third-stage larva. Most of the small strongyle species can only be identified as cyathostome parasites from the infective larval stage (Fig. 1.18 and Table 1.3). The posterior portion of the sheath of horse strongyle larvae is very long and filamentous, making these larvae easily recognizable as infective parasite larvae. Size is less helpful in distinguishing genera of these larvae. The number of intestinal cells in these larvae is variable and is useful in identification.

Fecal Egg Count Reduction Test

One of the principal uses of quantitative egg counts is the evaluation of drug efficacy. Anthelmintic resistance in strongylid nematodes of horses and small ruminants is rapidly increasing worldwide. While there are several techniques for evaluating anthelmintic efficacy, the only one currently practical for veterinary practitioners is the Fecal Egg Count Reduction Test (FECRT). In this procedure the percentage reduction in strongylid fecal egg counts following treatment is used to evaluate whether or not resistant worms are present.

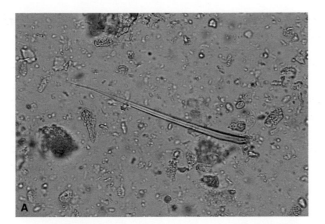

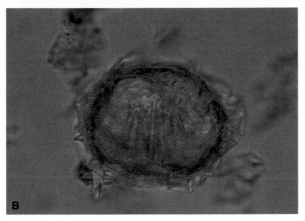

Fig. 1.11A and B. Examples of pseudoparasites. (*A*) Insect hair from the feces of an insectivorous bird. Insect and plant hairs may be confused with worms but have no internal structure. (*B*) This artifact in ruminant feces appears to have structures resembling the hooks of a tapeworm embryo, but there is no distinct embryo and the outer layer is poorly defined with projections that are variable in size and shape (40×).

To conduct the FECRT on a farm, 10–15 animals should be selected for an untreated control group and a similar number for each drug to be tested. Each animal used in the test should have a minimum of 150 strongylid eggs/g of feces. The Modified McMaster Test is the best technique for determining egg counts ranging from hundreds to thousands of eggs/g. If there is uncertainty about whether test animals will meet the 150 eggs/g minimum, it may be advisable to determine fecal egg counts from at least a portion of the test animals before doing the FECRT.

When performing the test, animals receiving anthelmintic treatment must be treated individually. The appropriate dose of drug must be determined for each animal and administered correctly. Alternatively, all animals can be given the dose of drug accurately determined for the heaviest animal in each group. Estimates of average weights must not be used for selecting a drug dose, since underdosing can reduce the efficacy of treatment even though worms are fully susceptible. Fecal samples should then be collected from all animals in the control and treatment groups 10–14 days after treatment and fecal egg counts determined. The percentage reduction in fecal egg counts is based on the formula

% reduction = $100(1 - [TM/CM])$

where TM is the mean egg count of the treated group and CM is the mean egg count of the untreated control group.

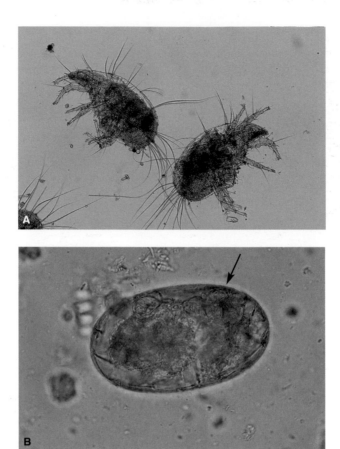

Fig. 1.12A and B. Examples of pseudoparasites. (*A*) Free-living mites that contaminate animal feed can be found in fecal flotation procedures. Unlike many parasitic mites, free-living species lack specialized structures on their legs (suckers, combs, etc.) for adhering to the host. (*B*) Eggs from free-living mites will also float in flotation solution. They are usually very large (>100 μm). Developing legs of the mite can sometimes be seen inside the egg (*arrow*).

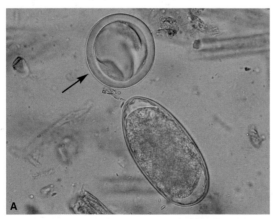

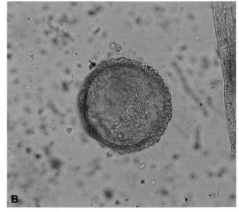

Fig. 1.13A and B. Examples of pseudoparasites. (*A*) In this ovine fecal sample both a strongylid egg and a pseudoparasite (*arrow*) are present. Characteristics helpful in recognition of pseudoparasites are lack of clear internal structure and discontinuities in the outer layer. (*B*) Pseudoparasite, probably a pollen grain (40×).

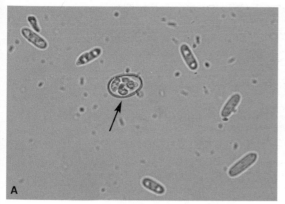 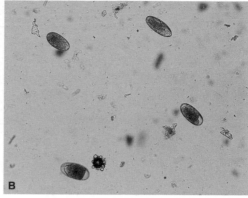

Fig. 1.14A and B. Spurious parasites are parasite eggs or cysts from another host that are acquired through predation or coprophagy and have merely passed through the digestive tract of the animal being tested. (*A*) Spurious parasites are common in samples from dogs that ingest fecal material. This *Eimeria* oocyst (*arrow*) is a typical spurious parasite in dog feces. It can be identified as *Eimeria* because it contains four sporocysts. Many *Eimeria* spp. oocysts also have a cap at one end. This photo also contains *Saccharomycopsis guttulatus,* a nonpathogenic yeast common in rabbits and seen occasionally in dogs (40×). (*B*) Eggs of livestock strongylid species can be found in feces of manure-eating dogs. Ruminant and equine strongylid eggs look like canine hookworm eggs but are larger.

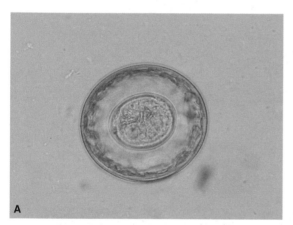 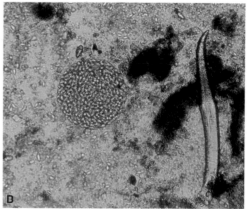

Fig. 1.15A and B. Examples of spurious parasites. (*A*) Tapeworm egg found in a fecal sample from a calf. Although the configuration of hooks inside this egg clearly identifies it as a tapeworm, it is most likely a rodent or bird tapeworm egg. (*B*) Cyst of *Monocystis,* a protozoan parasite of earthworms found in the feces of a snake that feeds on earthworms (10X).

A spreadsheet (RESO4) can be downloaded from the Website of the Australian Wool Initiative Limited (www.sheepwormcontrol.com) that will calculate the percentage reduction once the egg count data from each animal are entered. There is some variation in how the percentage reduction is interpreted depending on the host animal and the drug used. The RESO program utilizes guidelines that identify resistance when the percentage reduction is less than 95% and the lower 95% confidence interval is less than 90%, as recommended in Coles et al. 1992. However, for practical purposes, it is generally reasonable to suspect that some portion of the worm population is resistant if the percentage reduction is less than 90%. For example, if the percentage reduction is 10%, a large proportion of worms in the animals are probably resistant. If the reduction is 80%, the proportion of resistant worms is much smaller, but still significant. To further evaluate which worm species are resistant in ruminants, feces from both control and treatment groups can be cultured and the larvae

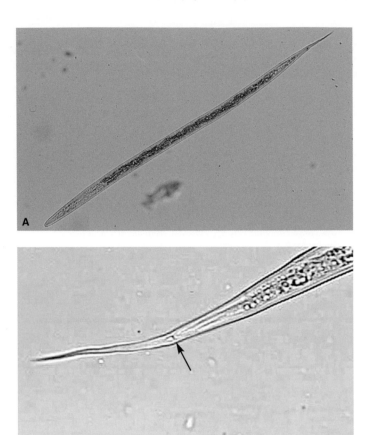

Fig. 1.16A and B. (*A*) Infective third stage of the ruminant strongylid parasite *Haemonchus*. (*B*) Posterior end of *Haemonchus* larvae. The cuticle of the second stage is retained as a sheath in the third-stage larva, and the length of the extension of the sheath beyond the tip of the tail (*arrow*) is used in identification. *Haemonchus contortus* larvae also show a slight kink in the sheath at the tip of the tail. Photo courtesy of Dr. Tom Yazwinski and Mr. Chris Tucker, Department of Animal Science, University of Arkansas, Fayetteville, AK.

identified (see above). In horses, drug resistance is present in small strongyles (cyathostomes), which cannot be differentiated to species with larval identification.

IDENTIFICATION OF ADULT WORMS

Tapeworm segments and adult gastrointestinal nematodes may occasionally be passed in feces and presented for identification by concerned owners. Segments of common tapeworms can usually be readily identified to the level of genus by shape and identification of eggs in the segments (see Figs. 1.74–1.75, 1.116 for photographs of common tapeworm segments), but nematode parasites may be more difficult to identify. When preserving nematodes for further identification, it is helpful to place them first in tap water and refrigerate the container for several hours. This will relax the worms and make them easier to examine. After relaxation, the worms can be placed in 10% buffered formalin. This is not the optimum preservative for all helminths but is readily available for most veterinarians.

The most common nematodes presented by pet owners are the ascarids (roundworms; see Fig. 1.45). These large, stout-bodied worms are common in feces and vomitus of kittens and puppies.

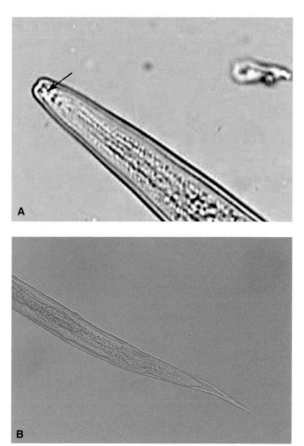

Fig. 1.17A and B. Features of infective third-stage trichostrongylid larvae: (*A*) Head of *Cooperia* sp. larva with two prominent refractile bodies (*arrow*). Photo courtesy of Dr. Tom Yazwinski and Mr. Chris Tucker, Department of Animal Science, University of Arkansas, Fayetteville, AK. (*B*) The end of the tail of *Trichostrongylus* larvae often shows one or two tubercles.

Equine owners might also see equine ascarids that are up to 50 cm (about 20 inches) in length. Smaller nematode worms present in equine manure may be the large and small strongyles or pinworms (*Oxyuris*). Larval or adult horse strongyles are usually red and no more than about 2–4 cm in length (see Fig. 1.129). *Oxyuris,* the equine pinworm, can reach 15 cm and the females have distinctive long, thin tails (see Fig. 1.135). Nematodes are most likely to be seen in diarrheic feces or following treatment.

Specific identification of adult nematodes is usually based on morphologic variations of the outer layer, or cuticle, of the worms. Microscopic examination of the mouthparts and accessory sexual structures may be required. To enhance visualization of these structures, the worm can be mounted in a clearing solution, which dissolves the soft tissue, leaving only the cuticle. If the worm is large, the areas of diagnostic importance (usually the anterior and posterior ends) can be cut off and mounted in a few drops of the clearing solution. Unfortunately, these solutions require either controlled or hazardous substances. Recipes for Hoyer's and Lactophenol solutions are given below but they are not usually prepared in veterinary practices. Depending on the species of parasite, accurate worm identification may require the evaluation of subtle morphological characteristics that will be unfamiliar to most practicing veterinarians. When specific parasite identification is needed, worms should be submitted to a parasitologist for examination.

Table 1.2. Morphologic characteristics of infective third-stage strongylid larvae of domestic ruminants

Genus	Overall Length (µm)	Anus to Tip of Sheath (µm)	End of Tail to Tip of Sheath (µm)	Other Characteristics
Trichostrongylus				
Sheep	622–796	76–118	21–40	Head rounded; tail of sheath short. Tail may
Cattle	619–762	83–107	25–39	have 1 or 2 tuberosities.
Ostertagia				
Sheep	797–910	92–130	30–60	Head squared; tail of sheath shorter in sheep.
Cattle	784–928	126–170	55–75	
Haemonchus				
Sheep	650–751	119–146	65–78	Head rounded; sheath tail medium length,
Cattle	749–866	158–193	87–119	offset.
Cooperia				
Sheep	711–924	97–150	35–82	Head squared with two refractile oval bodies
Cattle	666–976	109–190	47–111	at anterior end of esophagus; medium-length sheath tail tapering to fine point.
Nematodirus				
Sheep	922–1118	310–350	250–290	Broad, rounded head; intestine with 8 cells;
Cattle	1095–1142	296–347	207–266	tail notched and lobed; long thin sheath tail.
Bunostomum				
Sheep	514–678	153–183	85–115	Small larvae; rounded head; long thin sheath
Cattlle	500–583	129–158	59–83	tail.
Oesophagostomum				
Sheep	771–923	193–235	125–160	Rounded head; long thin sheath tail; 16–24
Cattle	726–857	209–257	134–182	triangular intestinal cells.
Chabertia				
Sheep	710–789	175–220	110–150	Rounded head; long thin sheath tail; 24–32 rectangular intestinal cells.

Sources: Bowman 2003; Ministry of Agriculture, Fisheries and Food 1986.

Hoyer's Solution

Hoyer's solution can be used indefinitely and a single recipe will last for many years. It also provides a permanent mounting medium for specimens, although the clearing process will continue until eventually internal structures will no longer be visible.

30 g gum arabic
16 ml glycerol
200 g chloral hydrate
50 ml distilled water

Dissolve the gum arabic in water with gentle heat. Add the chloral hydrate, then the glycerol.

Lactophenol

20 ml glycerin, pure
10 ml lactic acid
10 ml phenol crystals, melted
10 ml distilled water

Combine all ingredients.

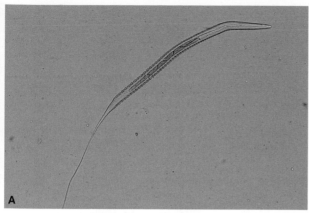
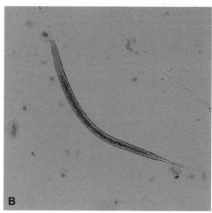

Fig. 1.18A and B. Infective third-stage larvae of both large and small equine strongyles have a very long filamentous extension of the sheath. (*A*) The larvae of small strongyles (cyathostomes) have 8 intestinal cells, which can be easily counted in the larva shown here. (*B*) Larvae of large strongyle species have more than 8 intestinal cells, like this *Strongylus vulgaris* larva with at least 28 cells.

Table 1.3.   Morphologic characteristics of infective third-stage strongylid larvae of horses

Genus	Characteristics
Strongyloides	Sheath absent; esophagus almost half the length of the body.
Trichostrongylus axei	Tail of sheath short, not filamentous.
Most small strongyles (Cyathostominae)	Long filamentous sheath; 8 triangular intestinal cells.
Gyalocephalus (small strongyle)	Long filamentous sheath; 12 rectangular intestinal cells.
Oesophagodontus (small strongyle)	Large larva; long filamentous sheath; 16 triangular intestinal cells.
Posteriostomum (small strongyle)	Long filamentous sheath; 16 roughly rectangular intestinal cells.
Strongylus equinus (large strongyle)	Long, thin larva; filamentous sheath; 16 poorly defined rectangular intestinal cells.
Triodontophorus (large strongyle)	Medium-length and broad larva; filamentous sheath; 18–20 well-defined rectangular intestinal cells.
Strongylus edentatus (large strongyle)	Smaller larvae; filamentous sheath; 18–20 poorly defined and elongated intestinal cells.
Strongylus vulgaris (large strongyle)	Large larvae; filamentous sheath; short esophagus; 28–32 well-defined, rectangular intestinal cells.

Note: Adapted from Ministry of Agriculture, Fisheries and Food 1986.

PARASITES OF DOMESTIC ANIMALS

The following photographs in this chapter illustrate the diagnostic stages found in feces of a wide variety of both common and some uncommon parasites of major domestic species. Because an appreciation of relative sizes of eggs, cysts, etc. is very helpful in identification, a line drawing precedes sections showing parasites of common mammalian hosts (Figs. 1.19 and 1.20). Generally, photographs of eggs and cysts were taken using the high-dry (40×) objective, although some photographs using the 10× objective are included to show relative sizes of eggs and cysts.

The figures in which each parasite appears are listed after the name. They may include figures in other sections where more than one parasite is illustrated.

An effort has been made to minimize taxonomic information while still permitting an appreciation of the larger groups to which each individual species belongs. For more specific taxonomic information, a textbook of veterinary parasitology should be consulted.

Helminth Ova and Protozoan Cysts
as found in freshly voided feces of the
Dog, Wolf, Coyote and Fox

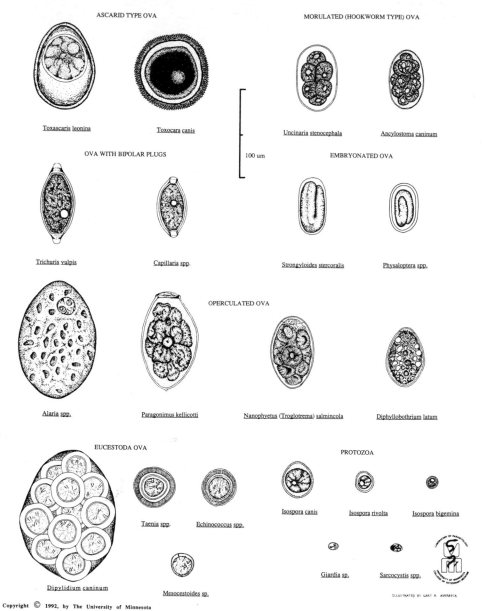

Fig. 1.19. Common parasites found in canine feces. Fig. courtesy of Dr. Bert Stromberg and Mr. Gary Averbeck, College of Veterinary Medicine, University of Minnesota, Minneapolis, MN. Note: *Isospora bigemina* is no longer a recognized species. *Neospora caninum* or *Hammondia heydorni* produce oocysts similar in size and appearance to *Isospora* oocysts.

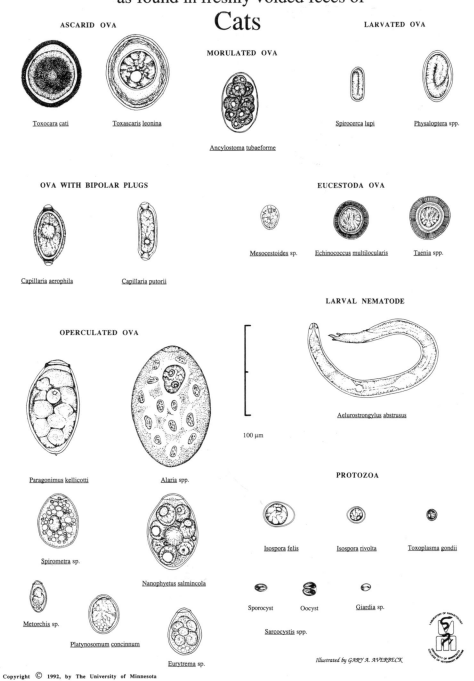

Helminth Ova, Larva, and Protozoan Cysts
as found in freshly voided feces of
Cats

ASCARID OVA

Toxocara cati

Toxascaris leonina

MORULATED OVA

Ancylostoma tubaeforme

LARVATED OVA

Spirocerca lupi

Physaloptera spp.

OVA WITH BIPOLAR PLUGS

Capillaria aerophila

Capillaria putorii

EUCESTODA OVA

Mesocestoides sp.

Echinococcus multilocularis

Taenia spp.

LARVAL NEMATODE

Aelurostrongylus abstrusus

100 μm

OPERCULATED OVA

Paragonimus kellicotti

Alaria spp.

Spirometra sp.

Nanophyetus salmincola

Metorchis sp.

Platynosomum concinnum

Eurytrema sp.

PROTOZOA

Isospora felis

Isospora rivolta

Toxoplasma gondii

Sporocyst

Oocyst

Giardia sp.

Sarcocystis spp.

Illustrated by GARY A. AVERBECK

Copyright © 1992, by The University of Minnesota

Fig. 1.20. Common parasites found in feline feces. Fig. courtesy of Dr. Bert Stromberg and Mr. Gary Averbeck, College of Veterinary Medicine, University of Minnesota, Minneapolis, MN. Note: Oocysts of *Hammondia hammondi* and *Besnoitia* spp. are similar in appearance to *Toxoplasma* oocysts.

Protozoan Parasites

PARASITE: *Isospora* **spp.** (Figures 1.21–1.25, 1.28, 1.44, 1.50, 1.70)
　　　　　Common name: Coccidia.

Taxonomy: Protozoan (coccidia). Several host-specific species are found in the dog (*I. canis, I. ohioensis, I. neorivolta, I. burrowsi*) and cat (*I. felis, I. rivolta*).

Geographic Distribution: Worldwide.

Location in Host: Small intestine, cecum, and colon.

Life Cycle: Cats and dogs are infected by ingestion of sporulated oocysts or transport hosts (rodents, etc). Following development in the final host, oocysts are passed in feces and undergo sporulation in the environment.

Laboratory Diagnosis: Oocysts are detected by centrifugal or simple fecal flotation examination. Oocysts have smooth, clear cyst walls, are elliptical in shape, and contain a single, round cell (sporoblast) when freshly passed.

Size:	*I. canis, I. felis*	38–51 × 27–39 μm
	other *Isospora* spp.	17–27 × 15–24 μm

Clinical Importance: These are the organisms typically referred to as "coccidia" of dogs and cats, although other parasites also fall into this taxonomic group. Oocysts can be found in the feces of many clinically normal young dogs and cats. Clinical coccidiosis most often occurs in puppies and kittens, often in association with weaning, change of owner, or other stress factors. Signs include diarrhea, abdominal pain, anorexia, and weight loss. In severe cases, bloody diarrhea and anemia may occur. Respiratory and neurologic signs have also been reported in some animals. Clinical disease has been difficult to reproduce in experimental infections.

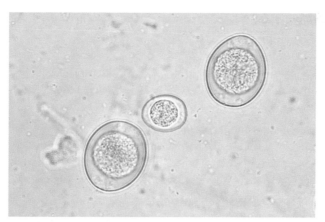

Fig. 1.21. Dog and cat coccidia species produce oocysts of different sizes. This Fig. shows *I. canis* (larger oocysts) and an oocyst of the *I. ohioensis* complex (smaller oocyst). Photo courtesy of Dr. David Lindsay, Virginia-Maryland Regional College of Veterinary Medicine, Virginia Tech, Blacksburg, VA.

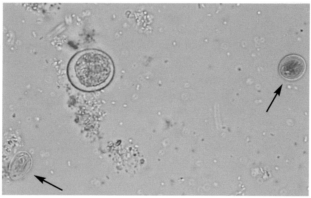

Fig. 1.22. *Isospora* oocyst and two iodine-stained *Giardia* cysts (*arrows*) in a canine fecal sample. Photo courtesy of Dr. Robert Ridley, College of Veterinary Medicine, Kansas State University, Manhattan, KS.

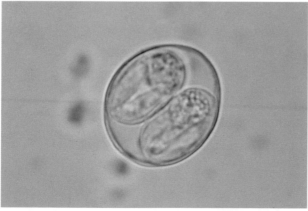

Fig. 1.23. Following passage in the feces, *Isospora* spp. oocysts undergo sporulation. The sporulated oocyst contains two sporocysts, each containing four sporozoites. Two sporozoites can be seen in each sporocyst of this oocyst, as well as the large, round residual body that is present in each sporocyst.

PARASITE: *Toxoplasma gondii, Neospora caninum* (Figure 1.26)

Taxonomy: Protozoa (coccidia).

Geographic Distribution: Worldwide.

Location in Host: Intestine and other tissues of cats and other felids (*Toxoplasma*) and dogs and other canids (*Neospora*).

Life Cycle: *Toxoplasma* is transmitted to cats by ingestion of cysts containing bradyzoites in tissues of intermediate hosts. Prenatal and transmammary transmission as well as direct transmission through ingestion of sporulated oocysts can also occur. Transmission of *Neospora* in dogs appears to be similar to *Toxoplasma* transmission.

Laboratory Diagnosis: Oocysts are detected in feces by centrifugal or simple flotation techniques. However, very few oocysts of *Neospora* appear to be produced in infected dogs. Serologic tests are available to identify current and past exposure to *Toxoplasma* in cats but are usually not positive until after fecal passage of oocysts has ceased. Dogs can also be tested for antibody to *Neospora*. The small, spherical-shaped oocysts of the two genera are morphologically identical, have a clear smooth cyst wall, and contain a single round sporoblast.

Size: 11–14 × 9–11 μm

Clinical Importance: *Toxoplasma* infections in cats are generally well tolerated. Clinical disease (ocular, respiratory, etc) can occur in cats, especially young or immunosuppressed animals. Toxoplasmosis is an important zoonotic disease with especially serious consequences in pregnant women and the immunosuppressed. Congenital *Neospora* infection can result in severe central nervous system disease in dogs. *Neospora* infection is also an important cause of abortion in the bovine intermediate host.

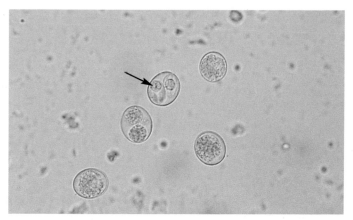

Fig. 1.24. *Isospora* oocysts usually require a minimum of 1–2 days to become infective for the next host (sporulated). In warm conditions, oocysts undergo the first cell division soon after being passed in the feces. In the two-cell stage they may be mistaken for sporulated oocysts. In this fecal sample a sporulated oocyst (*arrow*) is adjacent to one in the two-cell stage.

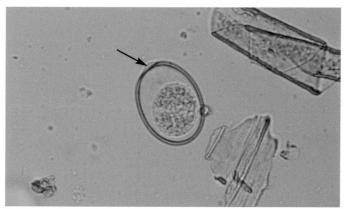

Fig. 1.25. *Eimeria* spp. oocysts are sometimes seen in dog and cat feces. *Eimeria* does not infect these hosts, but oocysts consumed as a result of predation or coprophagy will pass unharmed through the GI tract and may be misidentified as *Isospora*. Many (but not all) *Eimeria* oocysts have a knob at one end called the micropyle cap (*arrow*), whereas *Isospora* spp. lack a cap. If this cap is present, an oocyst in dog or cat feces can be identified as a "spurious parasite."

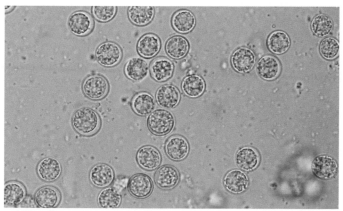

Fig. 1.26. *Neospora* and *Toxoplasma* oocysts are similar to common *Isospora* spp., but they are smaller. The oocysts of these two coccidia genera are similar in appearance and also cannot be distinguished from oocysts of *Hammondia*, another coccidian genus of small animals.

PARASITE: *Sarcocystis* spp. (Figures 1.27–1.28)

Taxonomy: Protozoan (coccidia). A number of species infect dogs or cats, each with a specific intermediate host.

Geographic Distribution: Worldwide.

Location in Host: Small intestine of dogs and cats.

Life Cycle: Cat and dog definitive hosts are infected by ingesting intermediate-host tissue containing sarcocysts. Sexual reproduction in dogs or cats leads to formation of oocysts that sporulate while still in the intestinal tract.

Laboratory Diagnosis: Oocysts form within the gastrointestinal tract of dogs and cats. The oocyst wall breaks down in the gut, and small, ellipsoidal sporocysts are released in the feces. They are detected by centrifugal or simple flotation techniques.

Size: 7–22 × 3–15 μm

Clinical Importance: *Sarcocystis* is generally nonpathogenic in the definitive host, although some species can cause severe disease in the intermediate host (cattle, sheep, pigs, horses).

PARASITE: *Cryptosporidium* spp. (Figure 1.29)

Taxonomy: Protozoan (coccidia). *Cryptosporidium felis* appears to be the primary species infecting cats, although *C. parvum* infection may occur in some cases. *Cryptosporidium canis* and *C. parvum* are found in dogs.

Geographic Distribution: Worldwide.

Location in Host: Small intestine.

Life Cycle: These parasites have a direct life cycle. Cats and dogs are infected following ingestion of oocysts, which are infective as soon as they are passed in the feces. Following asexual and sexual multiplication of the organism in the intestine, oocysts are produced and exit the host in the feces.

Laboratory Diagnosis: Small oocysts in the feces are detected by use of acid-fast or other stains of fecal smears, Sheather's sugar flotation test. Fecal antigen tests can also be used. Oocysts of *C. parvum* and *C. canis* are morphologically indistinguishable, while *C. felis* oocysts are smaller than those of the other two species.

Size: *C. felis*   3.5–5 μm in diameter
         C. parvum, C. canis   7 × 5 μm

Clinical Importance: Cryptosporidiosis has been reported as an uncommon cause of chronic diarrhea in cats. Affected cats are often immunosuppressed by other causes. *Cryptosporidium* infections in dogs and cats should be considered zoonotic, although the ease with which canine and feline species infect humans is still under investigation.

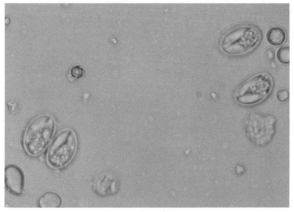

Fig. 1.27. *Sarcocystis* sporocysts are smaller than typical coccidia oocysts and have a smooth, clear cyst wall. Each sporocyst contains four banana-shaped sporozoites. Photo courtesy of Dr. Robert Ridley, College of Veterinary Medicine, Kansas State University, Manhattan, KS.

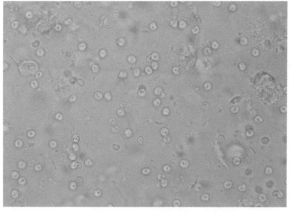

Fig. 1.28. *Sarcocystis* sporulates in the intestines and the oocyst wall usually ruptures before exiting the body so that only sporocysts are seen. Rarely, intact *Sarcocystis* oocysts are present (*arrow*). Large, round residual bodies can be seen in the sporocysts. This flotation preparation also contains an *Isospora* oocyst.

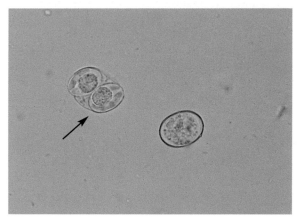

Fig. 1.29. *Cryptosporidium parvum* or *C. canis* in a sugar flotation preparation. The oocysts of these two species are indistinguishable by microscopic techniques; *C. felis* oocysts are slightly smaller in size. *Cryptosporidium* oocysts can also be detected with acid-fast stains and immunodiagnostic tests.

PARASITE: **Trichomonads** (Figures 1.30–1.31)

Taxonomy: Protozoan (flagellate). The species identification of these organisms in dogs and cats is currently under investigation. Recently, trichomonad organisms associated with chronic diarrhea in cats were identified as genetically identical to *Tritrichomonas foetus*, the cause of bovine venereal trichomoniasis.

Geographic Distribution: Probably worldwide.

Location in Host: Large intestine of cats and dogs.

Life Cycle: Very little is known about transmission. Infection is probably by direct contact since no environmentally resistant cyst stage is known to occur.

Laboratory Diagnosis: The presence of trophozoites can be detected in direct saline smears of fresh feces. Flotation solutions will destroy trophozoites. Trichomonad organisms can be confused with *Giardia* but have a rippling, undulating membrane and lack the facelike appearance of *Giardia* trophozoites. The InPouch® system used for culturing *Tritrichomonas foetus* infections in cattle (see Chap. 2) can also be used for diagnosis of feline trichomoniasis by adding 0.1 g or less of feline feces to the system and culturing at 25°C for up to 11 days (see Gookin et al. 2003).

Size: 6–11 × 3–4 μm

Clinical Importance: Cases of chronic diarrhea in cats have now been associated with infection; however, these organisms are generally considered to be of limited pathogenicity.

PARASITE: *Giardia duodenalis* (= *G. intestinalis*), *G. lamblia*, *G. canis*, *G. cati*, etc. (Figures 1.32–1.38, 1.22, 1.41)

Taxonomy: Protozoan (flagellate). The number and correct nomenclature of species are currently under investigation.

Geographic Distribution: Worldwide.

Location in Host: Small intestine of dogs, cats, many other animals, and humans.

Life Cycle: Dogs and cats are infected by ingesting cysts in the environment. Trophozoites are stimulated under certain conditions to encyst and are passed from the host in feces.

Laboratory Diagnosis: Examination of feces for cysts is the most sensitive microscopic technique. Cysts are best detected by 33% $ZnSO_4$ centrifugal flotation; other flotation solutions often cause rapid distortion. Motile trophozoites are occasionally seen in a direct saline smear of fresh diarrheic feces or may be in duodenoscopic aspirates (aspirates should be centrifuged and the sediment examined for trophozoites). Trophozoites are likely to be dead and unrecognizable if fecal examination occurs longer than 30 minutes after sample collection or if the sample has been refrigerated. Multiple fecal examinations (i.e., three exams done on samples collected over a 5- to 7-day period) may be necessary to rule out infection. Fecal EIA and IFA tests are also available.

Size: cyst   9–13 × 7–9 μm
           trophozoite   12–17 × 7–10 μm

Clinical Importance: *Giardia* is a common parasite of small animals. Many infections are asymptomatic, but *Giardia* may cause acute, chronic, or intermittent diarrhea, particularly in young dogs and cats. *Giardia* should be treated as a potential zoonotic organism; pets and livestock may be a source of environmental contamination and human exposure.

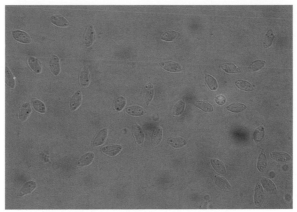

Fig. 1.30. Trichomonad parasites in dogs and cats have a distinctive undulating membrane. In fresh saline smears they are most easily confused with *Giardia* trophozoites, but trichomonads lack the facelike appearance and the concave ventral surface of *Giardia*.

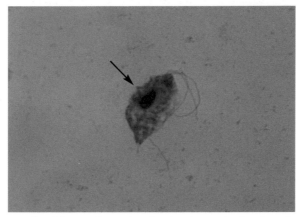

Fig. 1.31. Stained fecal smear of a trichomonad organism showing the anterior flagella and part of the undulating membrane (*arrow*).

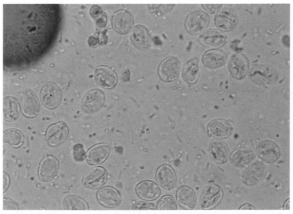

Fig. 1.32. *Giardia* cysts recovered with 33% ZnSO$_4$ centrifugal flotation. Cysts are elliptical with a thin, smooth cyst wall and contain two to four nuclei, two slender, linear intracytoplasmic flagella, and two thick, comma-shaped median - bodies.

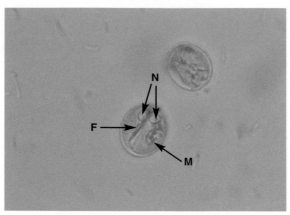

Fig. 1.33. A drop of Lugol's iodine may be added to a flotation preparation to stain *Giardia* cysts and make internal structures more prominent. Two nuclei (N), intracytoplasmic flagella (F), and median bodies (M) can be seen in the cyst shown here.

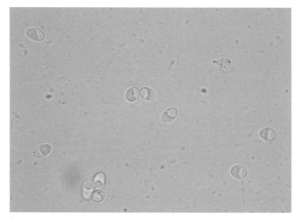

Fig. 1.34. *Giardia* cysts undergo osmotic damage when exposed to the high specific gravity of salt solutions. With time, increasing numbers of cysts appear vacuolated, with a characteristic half-moon shape. Plant pollen and yeast cells that mimic *Giardia* cysts do not undergo this same artifact change.

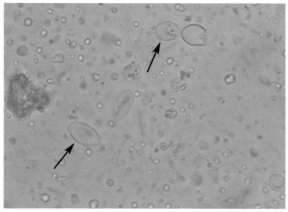

Fig. 1.35. The structures most often confused with *Giardia* cysts are yeast (*arrows*), which may be found in diarrheic feces in large numbers. Yeast are commonly slightly smaller than *Giardia* cysts and lack the complex internal structure seen in *Giardia* cysts.

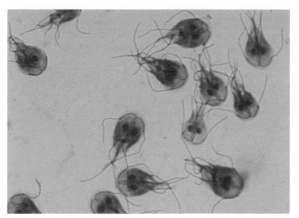

Fig. 1.36. Stained *Giardia* trophozoites in a direct smear. Trophozoites are bilaterally symmetrical and pyriform shaped with two nuclei, eight flagella, two rodlike median bodies, and a ventral, concave, adhesive disk that gives them a clown face.

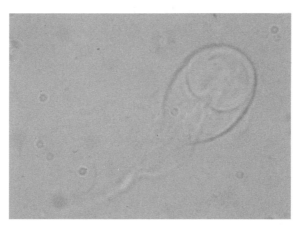

Fig. 1.37. *Giardia* trophozoite in an unstained smear. Live trophozoites have a characteristic wobbling motion when swimming (often described as looking like a falling leaf) and are easily kept in the microscope field of view.

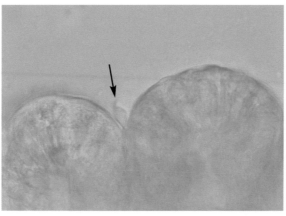

Fig. 1.38. *Giardia* trophozoite (*arrow*) associated with a portion of mucosa in a duodenal aspirate. Aspirates should be examined within 30 minutes of collection, before the fragile trophozoites die.

Helminth Parasites

PARASITE: *Ancylostoma* **spp.,** *Uncinaria stenocephala* (Figures 1.39–1.41, 1.44, 1.48–1.49, 1.80)
Common name: Hookworm.

Taxonomy: Nematodes (order Strongylida).

Geographic Distribution:
Ancylostoma caninum (dogs): worldwide; range in North America extends to southern Canada.
A. brasiliense (dogs and cats): tropical and subtropical distribution; in the USA found in the Gulf
Coast region.
A. tubaeformae (cats): worldwide.
A. ceylanicum (dogs and cats): various parts of Asia.
Uncinaria stenocephala (dogs, rarely cats): occurs in the cooler northern temperate regions, includ-
ing the northern USA, Canada, and Europe.

Location in Host: Small intestine of dogs and cats and wild canids and felids.

Life Cycle: Transmission of *A. caninum* to dogs occurs by transmammary transmission (most important), ingestion of infective third-stage larvae from the environment or in paratenic hosts, direct
skin penetration by infective larvae, and transplacental transmission (least important). Transmission
of *U. stenocephala* occurs by ingestion of infective third-stage larvae or paratenic hosts, and rarely
by direct skin penetration of infective larvae. Cats can be infected with hookworms either by skin
penetration by infective larvae or by ingestion of larvae in the environment or in paratenic hosts (rodents). Adult hookworms in the host small intestine produce eggs that exit the host in the feces.

Laboratory Diagnosis: Hookworm eggs are detected using centrifugal or simple flotation fecal examination techniques. *Ancylostoma* and *Uncinaria* eggs are morphologically identical, with an elliptical shape and smooth shell wall and containing a grapelike cluster of cells (morula). However,
they differ in size.

Size:	*Ancylostoma* spp.	52–79 × 28–58 μm
	U. stenocephala	71–92 × 35–58 μm

Clinical Importance: *Ancylostoma caninum* is common in North America. In heavy infections,
particularly in puppies, hookworms can cause severe anemia and death due to their voracious bloodsucking habits. Peracute, acute, and chronic disease syndromes may occur. *Ancylostoma brasiliense*
and to a lesser extent *A. caninum* pose a zoonotic risk (eosinophilic enteritis and cutaneous larva
migrans) to humans. *Ancylostoma* spp. infections in cats are less common than in dogs. Many feline infections are subclinical, but heavy infections causing anemia and weight loss can be fatal.
Uncinaria stenocephala is less pathogenic than *A. caninum*; infection may result in chronic disease
with diarrhea and hypoproteinemia.

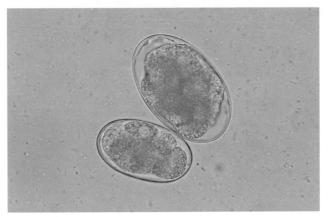

Fig. 1.39. Although *Ancylostoma* is the most common genus of hookworm in the USA, slightly larger *Uncinaria* eggs may also be seen in canine feces, and mixed infections can occur, as shown here.

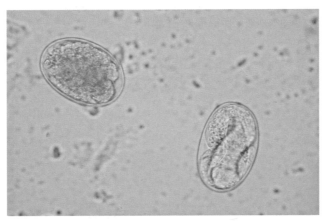

Fig. 1.40. *Ancylostoma tubaeformae* larvated and undeveloped eggs from a cat. The egg on the right contains a developed first-stage larva; the egg on the left is undifferentiated. Hookworm eggs exposed to warm temperatures for several hours rapidly develop to the larvated stage and hatch.

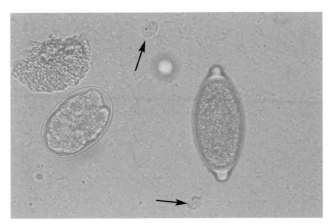

Fig. 1.41. Canine fecal sample containing *Ancylostoma caninum* (hookworm) and *Trichuris vulpis* (whipworm) eggs and two *Giardia* sp. cysts (*arrows*).

PARASITE: *Toxocara* **spp.** (Figures 1.42–1.47, 1.49, 1.70, 1.80)
Common name: Roundworm.

Taxonomy: Nematode (order Ascaridida).

Geographic Distribution: Worldwide.

Location in Host: Small intestine of dogs (*T. canis*) and cats (*T. cati*).

Life Cycle: Single-celled eggs pass from the host in the feces and develop to the infective stage in the environment. Dogs acquire infections of *T. canis* by transplacental (most important) and transmammary transmission or by the ingestion of larvated eggs or paratenic hosts (rodents). Cats acquire *T. cati* infection by transmammary transmission or ingestion of larvated eggs or paratenic hosts.

Laboratory Diagnosis: Eggs are detected using centrifugal or simple flotation examination techniques. *Toxocara* eggs have a dark, round, single-celled embryo contained in a thick shell wall. Eggs of the two species are difficult to differentiate. *Toxocara canis* tends to be subspherical, and *T. cati* elliptical in shape.

Size:	*T. canis*	85–90 × 75 μm
	T. cati	65 × 75 μm

Clinical Importance: *Toxocara* is an important pathogen in puppies and kittens. Stillbirths, neonatal deaths (*T. canis*), or chronic ill thrift (*T. canis, T. cati*) can occur in infected animals. Adult dogs and cats are much less likely to have symptomatic infections. Additionally, both species (especially *T. canis*) have zoonotic importance as causes of visceral and ocular larva migrans, particularly in children.

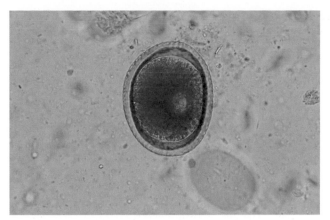

Fig. 1.42. *Toxocara* eggs are typical ascarid eggs with a thick shell. They contain a single cell when first passed in host feces.

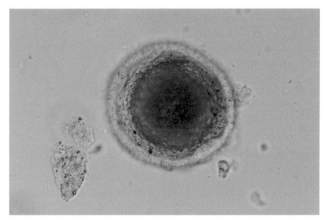

Fig. 1.43. When the microscope is focused on the surface of a *Toxocara* egg, the rough, pitted shell wall surface has a golf-ball-like appearance.

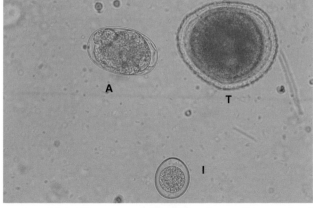

Fig. 1.44. Canine fecal sample containing *Toxocara canis* (T) and *Ancylostoma* (A) egg and an *Isospora* oocyst (I).

PARASITE: *Toxascaris leonina* (Figure 1.46)
          Common name: Roundworm.

Taxonomy: Nematode (order Ascaridida).

Geographic Distribution: Worldwide.

Location in Host: Small intestine of dogs, cats, wild canids, and felids

Life Cycle: The life cycle is similar to that of *Toxocara* spp., although there is no transmammary or transplacental infection. Dogs and cats are infected following ingestion of larvated eggs or paratenic hosts (rodents, rabbits).

Laboratory Diagnosis: Eggs are detected using centrifugal or simple flotation fecal examination techniques. *Toxascaris* eggs are elliptical with a thick, smooth outer shell wall containing a light-colored, single-celled embryo. The internal surface of the shell wall appears rough or wavy due to the vitelline membrane.

      Size: 75–85 × 60–75 µm

Clinical Importance: *Toxascaris* is much less common in dogs and cats than *Toxocara* and is considered to be of minor clinical significance.

PARASITE: *Baylisascaris procyonis* (Figure 1.47)
          Common name: Raccoon roundworm.

Taxonomy: Nematode (order Ascaridida).

Geographic Distribution: Parts of North America and Europe.

Location in Host: Small intestine of raccoons and occasionally dogs.

Life Cycle: Raccoons are infected by ingestion of infective eggs or paratenic hosts (rodents, rabbits, birds). Routes of infection in dogs are presumed to be the same.

Laboratory Diagnosis: Eggs are detected by simple or centrifugal fecal flotation examination. Eggs are thick walled, elliptical in shape, and contain a single, large, round-celled embryo. The eggs are often covered with a brown proteinaceous substance and have a fine granular shell wall surface.

      Size: 63–75 × 53–60 µm

Clinical Importance: Infection is well tolerated in the raccoon definitive host. Severe central nervous system or ocular disease can result from exposure of birds, rabbits, rodents, marsupials, and humans to infective *B. procyonis* eggs. Infections in dogs may result in either patent adult worms in the small intestine or larval tissue migration causing central nervous system disease.

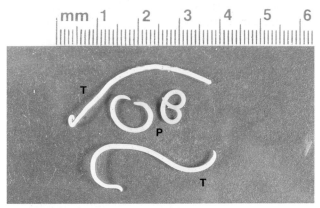

Fig. 1.45. Ascarids are often passed in the feces or vomitus of dogs and cats, particularly in young or recently dewormed animals. They are the only large, thick-bodied nematodes commonly seen by owners. Rarely, the stomach worm *Physaloptera* is present in vomitus. It usually assumes a C-shape when passed out of the host. Two specimens each of *Toxocara* (T) and *Physaloptera* (P) are shown here.

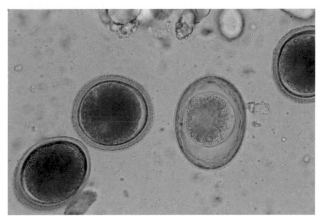

Fig. 1.46. *Toxascaris leonina* egg and *Toxocara cati* eggs. Note the dark single-cell embryo and rough mammillated (pitted) outer shell wall surface of the *Toxocara* egg contrasted to the lighter appearance of the embryo and to the smooth outer shell wall surface of the *Toxascaris* egg.

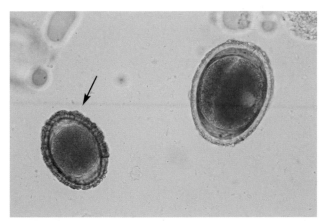

Fig. 1.47. *Toxocara canis* egg and *Baylisascaris procyonis* egg (*arrow*). *Baylisascaris procyonis* eggs appear in the feces of dogs due to either patent infections or coprophagy. The larger *Toxocara* egg (85–90 × 75 μm) has a rough, pitted, outer shell wall surface. The *B. procyonis* egg is smaller, has a finely granular shell wall surface, and may be brown in color. *Baylisascaris* eggs are easily misidentified as *Toxocara* in canine fecal exams. Mistakes can be minimized with the use of an ocular micrometer.

PARASITE: *Trichuris vulpis* (Figures 1.48–1.50, 1.41)
Common name: Whipworm.

Taxonomy: Nematode (order Enoplida).

Geographic Distribution: Worldwide.

Location in Host: Cecum and large intestine of dogs and wild canids. *Trichuris felis* infection has been reported rarely in cats in Latin America and Australia.

Life Cycle: Dogs are infected by ingesting infective eggs in the environment. Eggs are produced by adult worms in the large bowel and, after leaving the host in the feces, develop to the infective stage in the environment.

Laboratory Diagnosis: Eggs are best detected by centrifugal flotation and less effectively by simple flotation examination of feces. Eggs are typically symmetrical about the bipolar plugs, barrel shaped, and brown. The shell wall surface is smooth.

Size: 72–90 × 32–40 µm

Clinical Importance: Heavy infection in dogs can cause weight loss, unthriftiness, and a profuse diarrhea that may be bloody. Infection in humans occurs rarely.

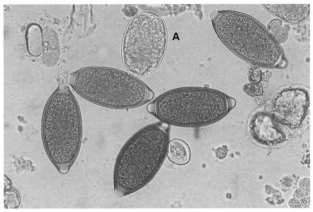

Fig. 1.48. The egg of *Trichuris vulpis* is one of the most common found in canine feces. The bipolar plugs are prominent and have ridges that give the appearance of being threaded into the shell wall. Capillarid species also produce eggs with similar polar plugs. In this fecal flotation preparation, an *Ancylostoma caninum* egg is also present (A).

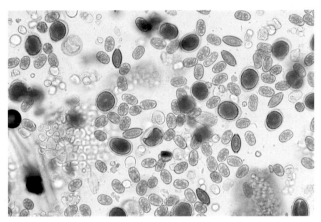

Fig. 1.49. *Toxocara, Ancylostoma,* and *Trichuris* eggs in a canine fecal sample. These are the most common intestinal helminths encountered in dogs. Photo courtesy of Dr. Robert Ridley, College of Veterinary Medicine, Kansas State University, Manhattan, KS.

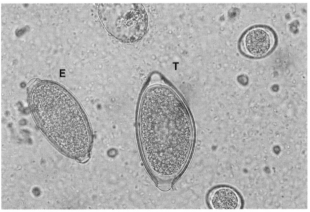

Fig. 1.50. The only canine parasite eggs that could be mistaken for whipworm eggs belong to the capillarid parasites *Eucoleus* and *Aonchotheca. Trichuris* eggs (T) are larger, have a smooth-walled shell, and are usually browner than the smaller *Eucoleus* egg (E) shown here. *Isospora* oocysts are also present in this sample.

PARASITE: *Eucoleus* (= *Capillaria*) *aerophilus, E. boehmi* (Figures 1.51–1.52, 1.50, 1.70)
Common name: Fox lungworm (*E. aerophilus*).

Taxonomy: Nematode (order Enoplida). These parasites were formerly in the genus *Capillaria* and are still frequently referred to by that name.

Geographic Distribution: *Eucoleus aerophilus* is found worldwide; *E. boehmi* has been reported from North and South America and Europe.

Location in Host: Trachea, bronchi, and bronchioles of dogs, cats, and foxes (*E. aerophilus*). Epithelium of the nasal turbinates and sinuses of dogs and wild canids (*E. boehmi*).

Life Cycle: The definitive host is probably infected by ingestion of eggs containing infective larvae, although an earthworm intermediate host may be involved.

Laboratory Diagnosis: Eggs are detected by fecal flotation examination or in tracheal or nasal mucus samples. The eggs are clear to golden (*E. boehmi*) or brownish green (*E. aerophilus*), are bipolar plugged, tend to be asymmetrical in shape, and contain a multicelled embryo.

Size:	*E. aerophilus*	58–79 × 29–40 µm
	E. boehmi	54–60 × 30–35 µm

Clinical Importance: *Eucoleus aerophilus* is an important pathogen in farmed foxes and causes bronchopneumonia. Infections in dogs and cats are usually subclinical; however, in some cases chronic cough occurs. *Eucoleus boehmi* infections are usually subclinical. Reported clinical signs include sneezing and a mucopurulent nasal discharge that may contain blood.

PARASITE: *Aonchotheca* (= *Capillaria*) *putorii* (Figures 1.53–1.54)

Taxonomy: Nematode (order Enoplida).

Geographic Distribution: North America, Europe, and New Zealand,

Location in Host: Small intestine and stomach of the cat, raccoon, and various wild felids and mustelids.

Life Cycle: Definitive hosts are infected following ingestion of larvated eggs. Adults develop in the gastrointestinal tract and produce eggs that are passed in the feces.

Laboratory Diagnosis: Eggs are detected by centrifugal or simple fecal flotation examination. The yellow-gray eggs are asymmetrical about the bipolar plugs. The sides of the eggs tend to be parallel. The shell wall surface has a network of deep longitudinal ridges.

Size: 56–72 × 23–32 µm

Clinical Importance: Infections in cats are usually subclinical and are uncommon in North America. Gastritis with vomiting can occur. Hemorrhagic enteritis can occur in mink.

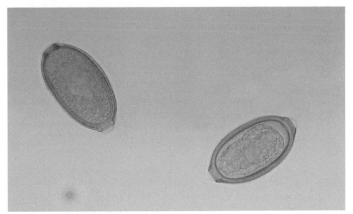

Fig. 1.51. *Eucoleus* eggs have bipolar plugs and may appear asymmetrical. Eggs are passed in the undifferentiated one- or two-celled stage. *Eucoleus boehmi* (*right*) and *E. aerophilus* (*left*) eggs are similar in appearance, although in fresh feces eggs of *E. boehmi* already contain a morula (cluster of cells) that does not completely fill the interior of the egg. Differences in the eggshell can also be used to differentiate the species (see Figs. 1.52, 1.54). Photo courtesy of Dr. Robert Ridley, College of Veterinary Medicine, Kansas State University, Manhattan, KS.

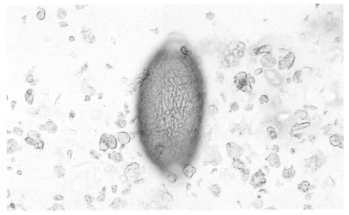

Fig. 1.52. Examination of the surface of the shell wall of small animal capillarid eggs can be used in making a specific identification. With the high-dry objective (40×) of the microscope, the surface of the *Eucoleus aerophilus* egg has a network of interconnecting ridges. The surface of the shell wall of *E. boehmi* (not pictured) is pitted, giving a stippled appearance.

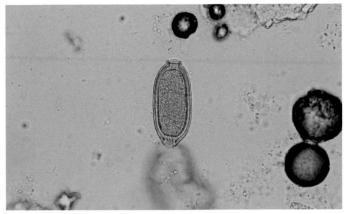

Fig. 1.53. Eggs of *Aonchotheca putorii* are similar to those of other capillarids.

Parasite: *Physaloptera* spp. (Figures 1.55–1.56, 1.45)

Taxonomy: Nematode (order Spirurida). Several species have been described (*praeputialis, felidis, pseudopraeputialis, rara, canis*).

Geographic Distribution: Worldwide.

Location in Host: Stomach of dogs, cats, and various wild animals.

Life Cycle: Cockroach, beetle, or cricket intermediate hosts ingest eggs shed in dog or cat feces. The definitive host is infected by ingesting the insect intermediate host or a paratenic host (reptiles and possibly other animals).

Laboratory Diagnosis: Eggs of this group of nematodes are not reliably detected by fecal flotation due to their density. *Physaloptera* eggs are best detected by fecal sedimentation. The eggs are clear and elliptical, have a smooth shell wall, and contain a larva coiled inside.

Size: 42–53 $\times$ 29–35 µm

Clinical Importance: This common parasite of several wild animal species is considered of minor clinical significance in dogs and cats. Infections may result in clinical signs of vomiting and anorexia.

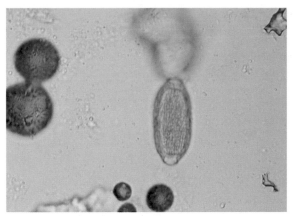

Fig. 1.54. In contrast to the ridges of the *Eucoleus aerophilus* egg, the shell surface of *Aonchotheca putorii* consists of a network of deep longitudinal ridges.

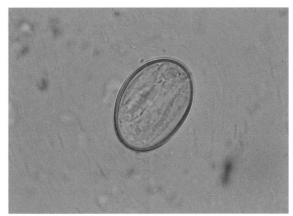

Fig. 1.55. *Physaloptera* eggs do not float consistently in routine flotation exams. The eggs are larger and less elongated than those of *Spirocerca* (Fig. 1.57). *Physaloptera* eggs are smaller and have a thicker shell than larvated hookworm eggs, with which they might be confused. Photo courtesy of Dr. Robert Ridley, College of Veterinary Medicine, Kansas State University, Manhattan, KS.

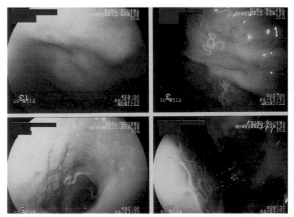

Fig. 1.56. Adult *Physaloptera* may be seen with gastroscopy in cases where routine fecal flotation does not detect the parasite eggs. Several worms can be seen on the surface of this canine stomach. Photo courtesy of Dr. Michael Leib, Virginia-Maryland Regional College of Veterinary Medicine, Virginia Tech, Blacksburg, VA.

PARASITE: *Spirocerca lupi* (Figure 1.57)
   Common name: Esophageal worm.

Taxonomy: Nematode (order Spirurida).

Geographic Distribution: Worldwide but primarily in warmer regions.

Location in Host: Adults are found in the wall of the esophagus, stomach, and, rarely, aorta of dogs, wild canids, and various other wild animals.

Life Cycle: Dung beetle intermediate hosts ingest eggs in feces. The definitive host is infected by ingesting the insect intermediate host or a paratenic host (rodents and various mammals, birds, reptiles).

Laboratory Diagnosis: Eggs are best detected by fecal sedimentation or (less reliably) by fecal flotation. The eggs are narrow, ellipsoidal, cylindrical, have a smooth, clear shell wall, and contain a fully developed larva coiled inside.

  Size: 30–38 × 11–15 μm

Clinical Importance: Infections are often subclinical. The most common clinical signs are dysphagia and regurgitation, but aortic stenosis, aneurysm, esophageal rupture or obstruction, cachexia, and esophageal sarcomas may occur. *Spirocerca* infection is uncommon in the USA.

PARASITE: *Angiostrongylus vasorum* (Figures 1.58–1.59)
   Common name: French heartworm.

Taxonomy: Nematode (order Strongylida).

Geographic Distribution: Canada (Newfoundland), Europe, South America, Africa.

Location in Host: Pulmonary arteries, right ventricle of dogs and foxes.

Life Cycle: First-stage larvae are passed in canine feces, and slugs and snails act as intermediate hosts of the parasite. Dogs and foxes are infected when they ingest intermediate hosts or paratenic hosts (frogs).

Laboratory Diagnosis: First-stage larvae in fresh feces are detected using the Baermann technique (most reliable) or fecal flotation. The larvae have a cephalic button on the anterior end, and there is a severe kink (S-shaped curve) in the tail, which has a dorsal spine.

  Size: 340–399 × 13–17 μm

Clinical Importance: The parasite is a serious pathogen of dogs, causing potentially fatal cardiopulmonary disease. Ocular and central nervous system disease and bleeding disorders have also been reported.

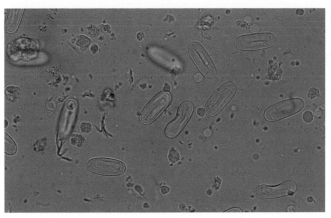

Fig. 1.57. *Spirocerca* eggs do not float consistently in common flotation solutions. These larvated eggs are more elongated than *Physaloptera* eggs. Photo courtesy of Dr. Isabella Verzberger, Atlantic Veterinary College, Charlottetown, PEI, Canada.

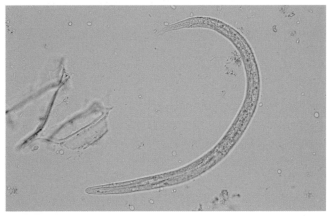

Fig. 1.58. *Angiostrongylus vasorum* first-stage larva. This species is uncommon in North America. Larvae can be differentiated from those of *Oslerus* in canine feces by the presence of the subterminal dorsal spine.

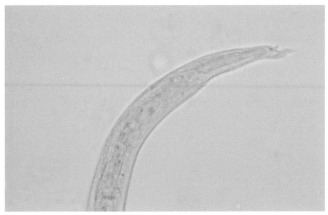

Fig. 1.59. High-magnification view of *Angiostrongylus vasorum* first-stage larva tail showing the S-shaped curve and the dorsal spine. The tail of *Aelurostrongylus abstrusus* (Fig. 1.60) is similar in appearance.

PARASITE: *Aelurostrongylus abstrusus* (Figure 1.60)

Taxonomy: Nematode (order Strongylida).

Geographic Distribution: Worldwide.

Location in Host: Lung parenchyma (terminal respiratory bronchioles, alveolar ducts) of cats and rarely dogs.

Life Cycle: First-stage larvae are released in the airways, coughed up, swallowed, and passed out in the feces. Cats are infected by ingesting a snail or slug intermediate host or paratenic hosts (rodents, birds).

Laboratory Diagnosis: First-stage larvae are detected in feces using the Baermann technique (most reliable) or by $ZnSO_4$ centrifugal flotation. The first-stage larval tail has a severe kink (S-shaped curve) and a dorsal spine.

Size: 360–400 $\times$ 15–20 μm

Clinical Importance: Infrequently diagnosed; infected animals may suffer signs of chronic cough and anorexia. Heavy infection may be fatal.

PARASITE: *Strongyloides stercoralis* (Figures 1.61–1.63)

Taxonomy: Nematode (order Rhabditida).

Geographic Distribution: Worldwide.

Location in Host: Adult females live in the canine small intestine.

Life Cycle: *Strongyloides* parthenogenetic females in the small intestine release larvae that may develop into infective parasitic larvae or, alternatively, may undergo a single free-living cycle of maturation and reproduction before infective parasitic larvae are formed. Infection of the host from the environment is primarily through skin penetration. Transmammary transmission may also occur.

Laboratory Diagnosis: First-stage larvae may be identified in fresh feces using a Baermann Test. *Strongyloides* larvae do not have the modifications of the tail seen in most lungworm larvae. They closely resemble hatched hookworm larvae or free-living nematodes that may be present in fecal samples that have been allowed to sit for a period of time prior to collection. If identification of the first-stage larvae is uncertain, larvae in the feces can be cultured for a few days and the third-stage larvae identified.

Size: 150–390 μm in fresh feces

Clinical Importance: Infections may be subclinical, but heavy infection can produce respiratory signs from migrating larvae as well as enteritis associated with adults. *Strongyloides stercoralis* also infects humans and may produce severe and even fatal infections in immunocompromised humans. The degree to which canine strains infect humans is unclear, but because of the seriousness of some human cases, infection in dogs should be considered a zoonosis.

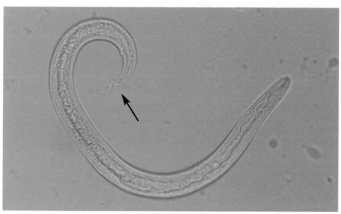

Fig. 1.60. *Aelurostrongylus* larvae have the S-shaped kink at the end of the tail that is typical of many members of this group of lungworms. These larvae also show a subterminal spine (*arrow*) that would not be present in other larvae found in feline feces. A higher magnification photo of a subterminal spine on a related parasite, *Angiostrongylus,* is shown in Fig. 1.59.

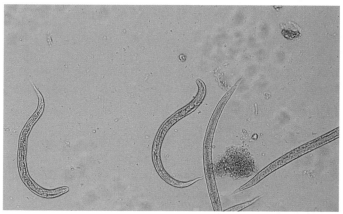

Fig. 1.61. *Strongyloides* first-stage larvae. In a fresh fecal sample *Strongyloides* larvae need to be differentiated from larvae of lungworm species. *Filaroides* and *Angiostrongylus* larvae have an S-shaped kink to the tail (see Figs. 1.59, 1.65). Larvae of *Crenosoma* can be differentiated from those of *Strongyloides* based on the morphology of the esophagus and tail (Fig. 1.64).

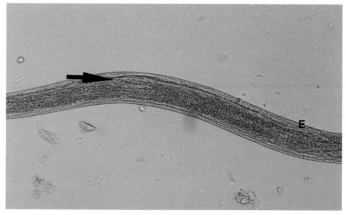

Fig. 1.62. A prominent genital rudiment (*arrow*) is also helpful in identifying first-stage *Strongyloides* larvae. The posterior end of the esophagus (E) can be seen in this portion of an iodine-stained larva.

PARASITE: *Crenosoma vulpis* (Figure 1.64)

Taxonomy: Nematode (order Strongylida).

Geographic Distribution: Northeastern North America and Europe.

Location in Host: Bronchioles, bronchi, and trachea of dogs, foxes, and various wild carnivores.

Life Cycle: Canid definitive hosts are infected by ingestion of slug/terrestrial snail intermediate hosts containing third-stage larvae. Larvae produced in the respiratory system by adult worms are coughed up, swallowed, and passed from the host in feces.

Laboratory Diagnosis: Detection of first-stage larvae in feces using the Baermann technique (most reliable) or by $ZnSO_4$ centrifugal fecal flotation. First-stage larvae tend to assume a C shape when they are killed by gentle heat or iodine. The terminus of the tail has a slight deflection but does not show the kink and spine seen in other nematode lungworms.

Size: 264–340 × 16–22 μm

Clinical Importance: *Crenosoma vulpis* infection in dogs produces a nonfatal chronic cough. Canine infection is generally rare in North America, excepting the Atlantic Canadian provinces, where crenosomosis is a frequent cause of chronic respiratory disease.

PARASITE: *Oslerus (= Filaroides) osleri* (Figure 1.65)

Taxonomy: Nematode (order Strongylida). Two other closely related species (*F. hirthi, F. milksi*) occur in the respiratory system of dogs but are rare and even more rarely cause disease.

Geographic Distribution: Worldwide.

Location in Host: Lumenal nodules in the tracheal bifurcation in dogs, coyotes, wolves, dingoes, and foxes.

Life Cycle: Infection follows ingestion of first-stage larvae from sputum or vomitus of an infected dog or other canid. This life cycle varies from that of other strongylid lungworms because the first larval stage is infective for the definitive host. Typically, the third larval stage is the infective form.

Laboratory Diagnosis: Diagnosis is best achieved by visual observation of the nodules on tracheal endoscopic examination. First-stage larvae may be detected in feces by $ZnSO_4$ centrifugal flotation or in transtracheal wash samples. The Baermann technique is *not* the method of choice because larvae passed in the feces are usually moribund or dead. The tail of the first-stage larvae has an S-shaped sinus wave curve but lacks a dorsal spine. The first-stage larvae of *O. osleri* are indistinguishable from those of *Filaroides hirthi*.

Size: larvae recovered from feces   232–266 μm
           larvae recovered from trachea   325–378 μm

Clinical Importance: This is an uncommon infection in dogs in North America. Younger animals tend to be more severely affected than older ones. Respiratory distress, chronic cough, and weight loss can occur. Heavily infected animals may die.

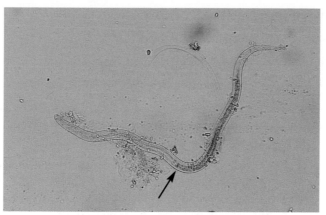

Fig. 1.63. To confirm identification of *Strongyloides stercoralis*, the fecal sample can be cultured for 2–4 days and examined for third-stage larvae, which have a characteristically long esophagus (*arrow indicates junction of esophagus and intestine*). Lungworm larvae will not undergo development in the fecal sample, and hookworm larvae require a longer period to reach the infective third stage.

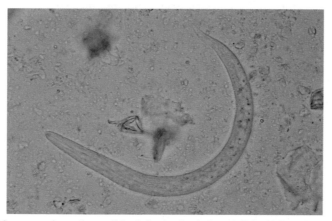

Fig. 1.64. The tail of *Crenosoma* larvae has a slight deflection but lacks a definite kink or dorsal spine, allowing it to be differentiated from *Aelurostrongylus, Angiostrongylus,* and *Oslerus*.

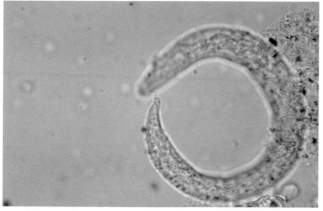

Fig. 1.65. First-stage *Oslerus* larva in dog feces. The larvae have a kinked tail but the accessory spine seen in *Aelurostrongylus* and *Angiostrongylus* larvae is not present. Photo courtesy of Dr. Jeffrey F. Williams, Vanson HaloSource, Inc., Redmond, WA.

PARASITE: *Ollulanus tricuspis* (Figure 1.66)

Taxonomy: Nematode (order Strongylida).

Geographic Distribution: Europe, North America, parts of South America, Australia.

Location in Host: Adult worms are found in the stomach of cats and other felids.

Life Cycle: Adult female worms in the stomach produce third-stage larvae that primarily leave the host in vomitus. Infection of cats occurs through ingestion of these larvae in vomitus.

Laboratory Diagnosis: Infection is diagnosed by identification of larvae or the small adults in vomitus, using a Baermann test. Rarely, stages of the parasite may be seen in feces, but they are usually digested before reaching the environment.

Size:	third-stage larvae	500 µm
	adults	700–1000 µm

Clinical Importance: Infection can cause chronic gastritis and vomiting in cats. Colony and feral cats are most often infected.

PARASITE: *Dipylidium caninum* (Figures 1.67–1.68, 1.71, 1.74–1.75)
        Common name: Double-pored or cucumber seed or flea tapeworm.

Taxonomy: Cestode.

Geographic Distribution: Worldwide.

Location in Host: Small intestine of dogs and cats.

Life Cycle: Animals acquire infection through the ingestion of larval cysticercoids contained in fleas or, less frequently, in chewing lice (*Trichodectes*, *Felicola*). Arthropod intermediate hosts become infected by the ingestion of egg packets/segments.

Laboratory Diagnosis: Tapeworm segments in the perianal area or in feces are often observed by owners. Specific diagnosis is made by identification of egg packets recovered from segments. Occasionally, eggs and/or egg packets are detected on fecal flotation examinations. Egg packets contain 2–63 eggs (average of 25–30 eggs).

Size:	egg packets	120–200 µm
	eggs	35–60 µm

Clinical Importance: Infections of this common tapeworm are generally subclinical; however, the passage of segments from the rectum may induce anal pruritis. *Dipylidium caninum* is zoonotic, with young children at greatest risk of acquiring infections from ingesting the infected flea or louse intermediate host.

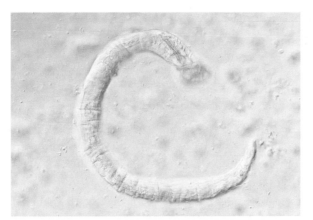

Fig. 1.66. Adult male *Ollulanus tricuspis* in a fecal sample. Larvae and adult worms are only rarely present in feces. Vomitus should be examined to diagnose infection. These worms can easily be differentiated from ascarids that may be vomited up by cats. The ascarid worms are several inches in length, while *Ollulanus* adults only reach a maximum length of 1 mm. Photo courtesy of Dr. Robert Ridley, College of Veterinary Medicine, Kansas State University, Manhattan, KS.

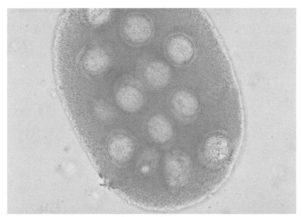

Fig. 1.67. *Dipylidium caninum* eggs containing a hexacanth embryo occur in packets of about 25–30 eggs. The hooks are readily visible inside the eggs shown here.

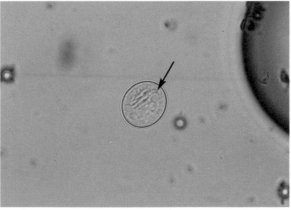

Fig. 1.68. Occasionally *Dipylidium* eggs are released from the packets and may be detected individually on fecal flotation. Note the clear, thin shell wall of the egg and the refractile hooks (*arrow*) of the embryo.

PARASITE: *Taenia* spp. (Figures 1.69–1.72, 1.74–1.75)

Taxonomy: Cestode. Numerous species infect small animals, including *T. taeniaeformis* in cats and *T. pisiformis, T. multiceps, T. hydatigena, T. ovis* in dogs.

Geographic Distribution: Worldwide.

Location in Host: Small intestine of dogs, cats, and various wild carnivores.

Life Cycle: Carnivores acquire infections through the ingestion of the immature metacestode stage (morphologic forms include cysticerci, coenuri, and strobilocerci) in the tissues of prey animals. Prey animals become infected with the metacestode through the ingestion of food contaminated with eggs passed in carnivore feces.

Laboratory Diagnosis: Eggs are detected when free in the feces by flotation techniques. Generally, however, eggs are passed from the host contained in tapeworm segments. Therefore, fecal flotation tends to be a poor indicator of infection status.

Size: 25–40 µm in diameter

Clinical Importance: Infections in the definitive host are generally subclinical; however, the passage of segments from the rectum may induce anal pruritis. *Taenia taeniaeformis* (small-rodent intermediate host) and *T. pisiformis* (rabbit intermediate host) are common species infecting pet cats and dogs, respectively. Metacestode infection in the intermediate hosts can cause disease (*T. multiceps*) or meat condemnation (*T. ovis*).

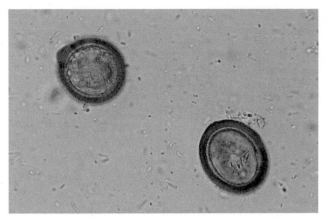

Fig. 1.69. *Taenia* eggs are brown with a thick shell wall (embryophore) and contain a hexacanth embryo (six hooks) Note the radial striations in the wall of the egg.

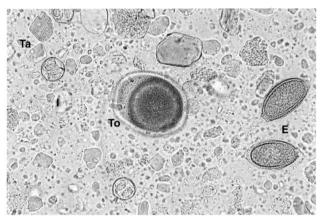

Fig. 1.70. Eggs of *Eucoleus* (E), *Toxocara* (To), and *Taenia* (Ta) and oocysts of *Isospora rivolta* (I) in a feline fecal sample. Photo courtesy of Dr. Robert Ridley, College of Veterinary Medicine, Kansas State University, Manhattan, KS.

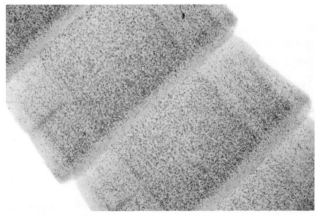

Fig. 1.71. Tapeworm segments from an animal can usually be easily identified as such by squashing the segment between two slides and identifying the eggs. Sometimes, however, segments are passed that contain no eggs. These can still be identified as segments by squashing them and observing the numerous small, round, transparent bodies, called "calcareous corpuscles."

PARASITE: *Echinococcus* spp. (Figures 1.72, 1.74–1.75)
Common name: Dwarf dog or fox tapeworm.

Taxonomy: Cestode. *Echinococcus granulosus* and *E. multilocularis* infect dogs and wild canids. Cats are infrequently infected with *E. multilocularis.*

Geographic Distribution: *Echinococcus granulosus* is found worldwide, *E. multilocularis* occurs in the USA, Canada, and in parts of Europe and Asia.

Location in Host: Small intestine.

Life Cycle: Carnivores acquire infections through the ingestion of metacestodes (hydatids) in the tissues of prey animals. Prey animals become infected with the metacestode through the ingestion of eggs passed in carnivore feces.

Laboratory Diagnosis: Like the eggs of *Taenia*, *Echinococcus* eggs have a thick shell wall with radial striations (embryophore). The 6 hooks of the hexacanth embryo allow it to be distinguished from pollen grains or other debris. The eggs of *Taenia* and *Echinococcus* are morphologically identical.

Size: 25–40 μm in diameter

Clinical Importance: Infections in the definitive host are subclinical. *Echinococcus* spp. are important due to their zoonotic potential. Human infection with hydatid cysts can cause serious disease and death. In some countries, particularly in rural areas, hydatid disease can be an important public health problem. In most areas of North America, canine infection and human hydatid disease are rare.

PARASITE: *Mesocestoides* spp. (Figures 1.73–1.75)

Taxonomy: Cestode. Species include *M. corti, M. lineatus, M. variabilis.*

Geographic Distribution: Worldwide.

Location in Host: Small intestine of dogs, cats, various wild mammals, and birds.

Life Cycle: The life cycle is not completely known. Dogs and cats acquire infections through ingestion of tetrathyridia contained in the tissues of various reptiles, amphibia, birds, and mammal intermediate hosts. Eggs are passed in motile segments in the feces of infected dogs and cats. The first intermediate host and the form of the first larval stage of *Mesocestoides* are unknown.

Laboratory Diagnosis: Club-shaped segments are passed in the feces. Eggs are contained in a round parauterine organ at the broad end of the segment. Eggs are rarely found free in the feces of definitive hosts but would, presumably, be detected by fecal flotation.

Size: eggs 30–40 μm in diameter

Clinical Importance: Infection of the definitive host with the adult tapeworm is usually subclinical. Fatal peritonitis due to large numbers of tetrathyridia or acephalic metacestodes has been reported in dogs acting as hosts to the larval stages.

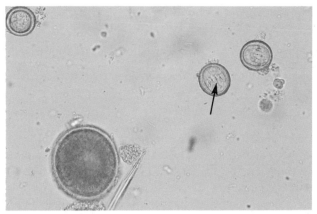

Fig. 1.72. Embryonic hooks are clearly visible in the two *Taenia* or *Echinococcus* eggs in this photo (*arrow*). Hooks can be used to differentiate tapeworm eggs from similar artifacts like pollen grains. The eggs of *Taenia* and *Echinococcus* are morphologically identical. A *Toxocara* egg is also present.

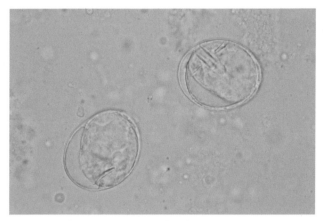

Fig. 1.73. *Mesocestoides* eggs have a thin, clear, smooth shell wall and contain a hexacanth embryo. The hooks of the embryo are readily visible.

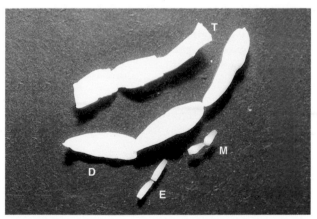

Fig. 1.74. Mature tapeworm segments passed in the feces may be observed by owners and presented for identification. The size and shape of these segments are quite characteristic: *Taenia* segments (T) are square to rectangular in shape, *Dipylidium* segments (D) are more barrel shaped, and *Mesocestoides* has club-shaped segments (M). Both *Mesocestoides* and *Echinococcus* (E) segments are small and are often overlooked. Identification can be confirmed by examining eggs from the segments.

PARASITE: *Diphyllobothrium latum* (Figure 1.76)
        Common name: Broad fish tapeworm.

Taxonomy: Cestode. Dogs and cats can also be infected with *D. dendriticum* and *D. ditremum*.

Geographic Distribution: Northern Hemisphere and South America.

Location in Host: Small intestine of dogs, cats, pigs, humans, and various other fish-eating mammals.

Life Cycle: Eggs passed in the feces of the final host hatch coracidia, which are ingested by freshwater copepods (first intermediate hosts). Fish eat the copepods containing the next larval stage (procercoids), which develop into the plerocercoids (infective stage) in the fish. Predatory fish can acquire plerocercoids through ingestion of infected smaller fish. Mammalian definitive hosts acquire infections through the ingestion of plerocercoids contained in the tissues of fish.

Laboratory Diagnosis: The eggs can be detected in feces using a sedimentation technique. Lengths of reproductively spent segments are occasionally passed in the feces.

    Size: eggs 58–76 × 40–51 μm

Clinical Importance: Uncommon in pets in North America. Infections are generally subclinical in dogs and cats. Dogs and cats do not serve as direct sources of infection for humans. Human infection with this tapeworm may lead to the development of vitamin B12 deficiency.

PARASITE: *Spirometra* spp. (Figure 1.77)
        Common name: Zipper tapeworm.

Taxonomy: Cestode.

Geographic Distribution: *Spirometra mansonoides* occurs in North and South America, and *S. erinaceieuropaei* occurs in Europe and Asia.

Location in Host: Small intestine of cats, dogs, and wild animals.

Life Cycle: Dogs and cats acquire infections by the ingestion of frogs, snakes, rodents, or birds containing plerocercoids (known as spargana). Eggs passed in the feces of dogs and cats hatch coracidia, which are eaten by freshwater copepods and develop into procercoids. The second intermediate hosts (frogs, snakes, etc.) acquire plerocercoids by feeding on the copepods.

Laboratory Diagnosis: The yellow-brown eggs can be detected in feces using a sedimentation technique but are also often recovered in flotation procedures. Lengths of reproductively spent segments are occasionally passed in the feces.

    Size: eggs 65–70 × 35–37 μm

Clinical Importance: Infections in the definitive hosts are usually subclinical. Cats can also serve as a paratenic host, with plerocercoids surviving in various tissues (sparganosis) and causing clinical signs depending on their location.

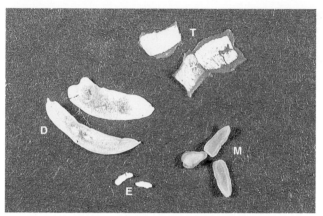

Fig. 1.75. Within hours of passing from the host, tapeworm segments lose their motility and dry up. Clients may find dried tapeworm segments in resting areas of dogs and cats. The dried segments still retain their characteristic shape. Shown in this photo are *Taenia* (T), *Echinococcus* (E), *Dipylidium* (D), and *Mesocestoides* (M) segments.

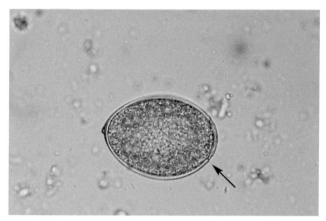

Fig. 1.76. Unlike common tapeworms, *Diphyllobothrium* eggs lack hooks and resemble trematode eggs. They are light brown with a cap (operculum) at one end (*arrow*). They contain an undifferentiated embryo surrounded by yolk cells that completely fill the space within the eggshell. A pore in the shell wall at the pole opposite to the operculum is often visible due to the slight bit of protein protruding from it.

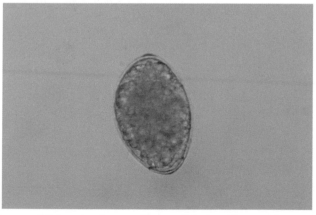

Fig. 1.77. The operculate eggs of *Spirometra* also resemble trematode eggs. They contain an undifferentiated embryo and yolk cells that completely fill the space within the eggshell. The eggs are asymmetrical about the long axis.

PARASITE: *Alaria* spp. (Figures 1.78–1.80)

Taxonomy: Trematode.

Geographic Distribution: Worldwide.

Location in Host: Small intestine of dogs, cats, and various wild carnivores.

Life Cycle: Eggs are passed in the feces of the mammalian host. Following larval development in a snail intermediate host, a second intermediate host (frog) is infected. Infection of dogs and cats occurs by ingestion of frogs or various paratenic hosts harboring the larval stage (mesocercaria). Transmammary transmission has been reported in cats.

Laboratory Diagnosis: The most reliable method is detection of eggs by sedimentation examination of feces, although sometimes eggs may be detected on fecal flotation.

    Size: 98–134 × 62–68 μm

Clinical Importance: Infections are generally nonpathogenic in dogs and cats. *Alaria* is a potentially serious zoonotic risk to humans through the ingestion of raw or improperly cooked frogs containing mesocercaria.

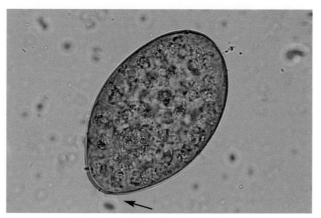

Fig. 1.78. *Alaria* eggs are large, operculate, and yellow-brown and contain an undifferentiated embryo surrounded by yolk cells. The operculum in this egg is difficult to see but is marked by a discontinuity in the shell (*arrow*).

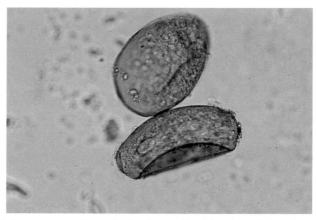

Fig. 1.79. Sometimes *Alaria* spp. eggs are detected using the centrifugal flotation technique; however, egg morphology may be altered: the eggs appear collapsed or folded due to the osmotic pressure associated with the high specific gravity of the flotation solution

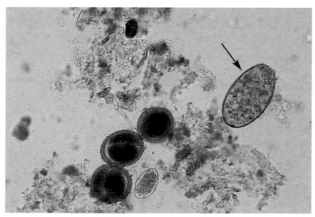

Fig. 1.80. The large size of *Alaria* spp. eggs is evident in this fecal sample containing eggs of *Alaria* (*arrow*), *Toxocara*, and *Ancylostoma*.

PARASITE: *Paragonimus kellicotti* (Figure 1.81)

Taxonomy: Trematode.

Geographic Distribution: North America. Other, similar species of *Paragonimus* that infect domestic animals, humans and wildlife occur in South and Central America, Africa, and Asia.

Location in Host: Lung parenchyma of cats, dogs, pigs, goats, minks, and various other wild mammals.

Life Cycle: Snails are infected by the larval stage emerging from eggs released in the feces of definitive hosts. Crayfish serve as the second intermediate hosts. Dogs and cats acquire infection by ingesting the metacercaria in the tissues of crayfish or paratenic hosts.

Laboratory Diagnosis: A sedimentation technique (recommended) or fecal flotation (less reliable) can be used to detect the yellow-brown, operculate eggs, which have a thickened ridge in the shell wall along the line of the operculum.

Size: 75–118 × 42–67 μm

Clinical Importance: Infection may be subclinical or cause eosinophilic bronchitis and granulomatous pneumonia, resulting in chronic cough and lethargy. Infections can be fatal.

PARASITE: *Heterobilharzia americana* (Figures 1.82–1.83)

Taxonomy: Trematode.

Geographic Distribution: Southeastern USA.

Location in Host: Mesenteric and hepatic portal veins of dogs and various wildlife species.

Life Cycle: Eggs released in the feces of dogs produce ciliated larvae (miracidia) that develop in a snail intermediate host. Cercariae that are released from the snail intermediate host infect dogs and wildlife through direct skin penetration.

Laboratory Diagnosis: Eggs can be detected by sedimentation examination of feces in saline (or 5% formol-saline). It is important to use saline in the procedure because eggs are stimulated to hatch when they contact water. The free-swimming miracidia larvae can be observed by placing the sediment in water after performing the sedimentation procedure with saline.

Size: eggs 74–113 × 60–80 μm

Clinical Importance: Infection with *H. americana* in dogs is uncommon in most areas. Infection can cause chronic diarrhea, anorexia, and emaciation. *Heterobilharzia* also has zoonotic importance as one of the causal agents of cercarial dermatitis (Swimmer's Itch) in humans.

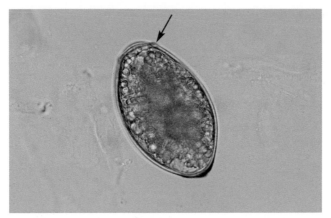

Fig. 1.81. *Paragonimus* eggs are undifferentiated when passed in the feces. The yellow-brown, operculate eggs can be differentiated by the characteristic thickened ridge in the shell wall along the line of the operculum (*arrow*). Collapsed eggs may be seen in flotation preparations.

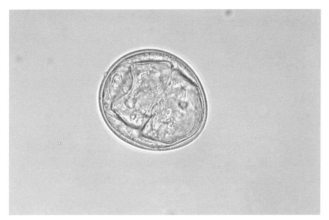

Fig. 1.82. The large, elliptical eggs of *Heterobilharzia americana* have a smooth, thin shell wall and contain a fully formed miracidium. The shell wall of the egg lacks an operculum. Photo courtesy of Dr. Bruce Hammerberg and Dr. James Flowers, College of Veterinary Medicine, North Carolina State University, Raleigh, NC.

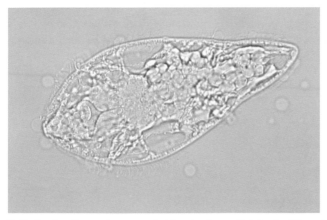

Fig. 1.83. On contact with freshwater, *H. americana* eggs hatch, releasing a ciliated miracidium stage. To prevent hatching of the eggs, a sedimentation procedure for diagnosis should be performed using saline instead of water. Photo courtesy of Dr. Bruce Hammerberg and Dr. James Flowers, College of Veterinary Medicine, North Carolina State University, Raleigh, NC.

PARASITE: *Nanophyetus salmincola* (Figure 1.84)
Common name: Salmon poisoning fluke.

Taxonomy: Trematode.

Geographic Distribution: Pacific Northwest region of North America.

Location in Host: Small intestine of dogs, cats, and various other piscivorous carnivores.

Life Cycle: Dogs and cats are infected by the ingestion of metacercaria in the tissues of salmonid fish (second intermediate hosts). Snails serve as the first intermediate host.

Laboratory Diagnosis: Eggs can be detected by sedimentation examination of feces.

Size: 72–97 × 35–55 μm

Clinical Importance: *Nanophyetus salmincola* serves as a vector for the causal agent of Salmon Poisoning Disease (*Neorickettsia helminthoeca*) and Elokomin Fluke Fever (*Neorickettsia* sp.). Salmon Poisoning Disease is extremely pathogenic in dogs.

PARASITE: *Platynosomum concinnum* (Figures 1.85–1.86)

Taxonomy: Trematode.

Geographic Distribution: Southeastern USA, South America, West Africa. Other flukes that may be found in the bile or pancreatic ducts in North America include *Eurytrema procyonis* and *Fasciola hepatica*.

Location in Host: Gall bladder and bile ducts of cats.

Life Cycle: Adult worms produce eggs that are passed in the feces of cats. The life cycle is complex, involving snail, crustacean, and amphibian or reptile intermediate hosts. Cats are infected following ingestion of lizards or amphibians containing larvae.

Laboratory Diagnosis: A sedimentation procedure is most effective for recovering the relatively small, operculate eggs of *Platynosomum*.

Size: 34–50 × 20–35 μm

Clinical Significance: Light infections are asymptomatic. Heavily infected cats may show signs of weight loss and hepatomegaly.

Dogs and cats may also rarely be infected with acanthocephalan (*Onicola, Macracanthorhynchus*) and pentastomid (*Linguatula*) parasites. Eggs of parasites belonging to these groups are shown in Figures 1.152 and 1.199.

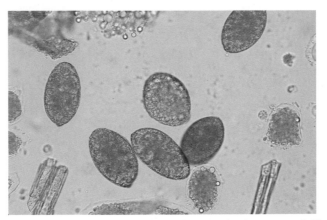

Fig. 1.84. The operculated eggs of *Nanophyetus* contain an undifferentiated embryo surrounded by yolk cells.

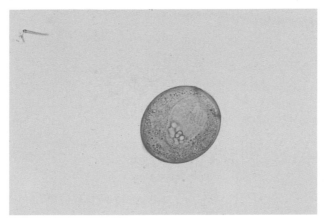

Fig. 1.85. The small brown eggs of *Platynosomum* have an operculum at one end and are unlikely to be seen with routine flotation procedures. Photo courtesy of Dr. Robert Ridley, College of Veterinary Medicine, Kansas State University, Manhattan, KS.

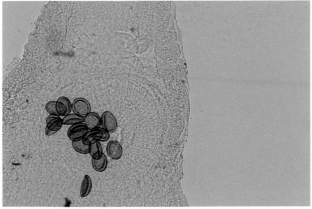

Fig. 1.86. Cats in the eastern USA are rarely infected with the pancreatic fluke *Eurytrema procyonis* and their eggs may be detected in feces. Small brown eggs can be seen within the body of this adult pancreatic fluke.

Helminth Ova, Larva and Protozoan Cysts
as found in freshly voided feces of
Cattle

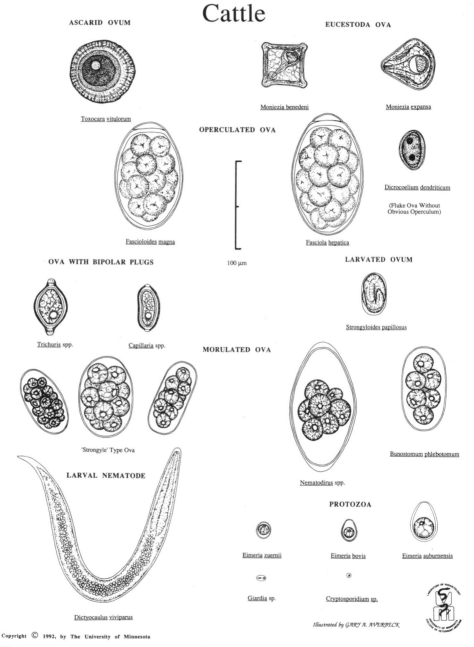

ASCARID OVUM

Toxocara vitulorum

EUCESTODA OVA

Moniezia benedeni

Moniezia expansa

OPERCULATED OVA

Dicrocoelium dendriticum

(Fluke Ova Without Obvious Operculum)

Fascioloides magna

Fasciola hepatica

OVA WITH BIPOLAR PLUGS

100 μm

LARVATED OVUM

Strongyloides papillosus

Trichuris spp.

Capillaria spp.

MORULATED OVA

'Strongyle' Type Ova

LARVAL NEMATODE

Bunostomum phlebotomum

Nematodirus spp.

PROTOZOA

Eimeria zuernii

Eimeria bovis

Eimeria auburnensis

Giardia sp.

Cryptosporidium sp.

Dictyocaulus viviparus

Illustrated by GARY A. AVERBECK

Copyright © 1992, by The University of Minnesota

Fig. 1.87. Common parasites found in bovine feces. Fig. courtesy of Dr. Bert Stromberg and Mr. Gary Averbeck, College of Veterinary Medicine, University of Minnesota, Minneapolis, MN.

Helminth Ova, Larva and Protozoan Cysts
as found in freshly voided feces of
Sheep and Goats

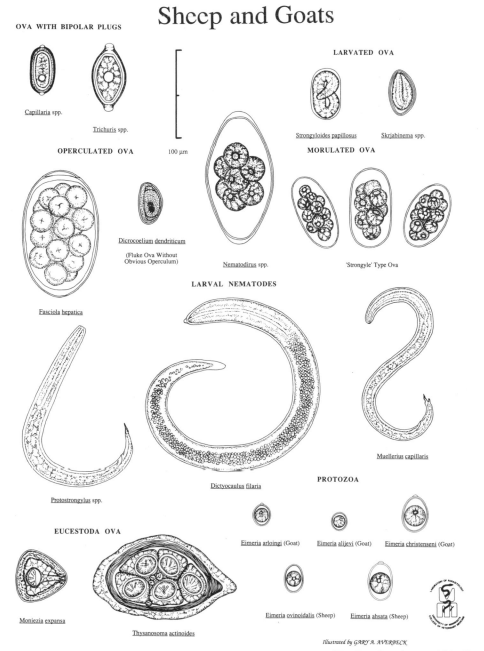

OVA WITH BIPOLAR PLUGS

Capillaria spp.

Trichuris spp.

100 μm

LARVATED OVA

Strongyloides papillosus

Skrjabinema spp.

OPERCULATED OVA

Dicrocoelium dendriticum

(Fluke Ova Without Obvious Operculum)

Nematodirus spp.

MORULATED OVA

'Strongyle' Type Ova

Fasciola hepatica

LARVAL NEMATODES

Muellerius capillaris

Dictyocaulus filaria

Protostrongylus spp.

PROTOZOA

EUCESTODA OVA

Eimeria arloingi (Goat)

Eimeria alijevi (Goat)

Eimeria christenseni (Goat)

Eimeria ovinoidalis (Sheep)

Eimeria ahsata (Sheep)

Moniezia expansa

Thysanosoma actinoides

Illustrated by GARY A. AVERBECK

Fig. 1.88. Common parasites found in feces of sheep and goats. Fig. courtesy of Dr. Bert Stromberg and Mr. Gary Averbeck, College of Veterinary Medicine, University of Minnesota, Minneapolis, MN.

Protozoan Parasites

PARASITE: *Eimeria* **spp.** (Figures 1.89–1.92, 1.101, 1.105)
Common name: Coccidia.

Taxonomy: Protozoan (coccidia).

Geographic Distribution: Worldwide.

Location in Host: Many host-specific species of *Eimeria* infect the intestinal tract of domestic ruminants and camelids.

Life Cycle: Fecal oocysts sporulate in the environment and infect intestinal cells following ingestion. Asexual and sexual reproduction is followed by the production of oocysts that exit the host in manure. Sporulated oocysts can survive for long periods under favorable environmental conditions.

Laboratory Diagnosis: Oocysts are found on routine fecal flotation exam. Species identification is difficult and, in most cases, requires microscopic exam of sporulated (infective) oocysts. Although the number of oocysts in the feces has been used as an indicator of clinical disease, high numbers of oocysts can also be present in the absence of clinical signs.

Size: approx. 12–45 μm in length (oocyst), depending on species

Clinical Importance: Most ruminants become infected with coccidia at an early age, and low-level infection persists through adulthood. While infection is often subclinical, coccidiosis is a common cause of diarrhea in young ruminants. Signs range from mild diarrhea to severe, bloody diarrhea.

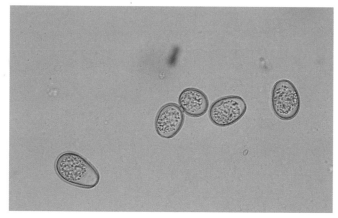

Fig. 1.89. *Eimeria* spp. oocysts have a thin wall and are oval or round. When seen in fresh feces, oocysts contain a single cell.

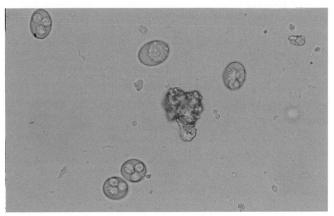

Fig. 1.90. *Eimeria* oocysts undergo sporulation in the environment, resulting in an infective oocyst that contains four sporocysts, each containing two sporozoites. Four of the oocysts in this sample are in the four-cell stage, which precedes the development of sporocysts.

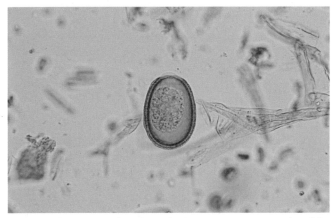

Fig. 1.91. One of the most distinctive oocysts of ruminants is *Eimeria intricata*, a parasite of sheep. The oocyst is brown and larger than other ovine *Eimeria*. The micropyle cap at the end of the oocyst is easily seen in this specimen. This cap occurs in many, but not all, *Eimeria* spp. and is helpful in identifying the genus in dogs that have eaten manure and are passing oocysts from horses or ruminants in their feces.

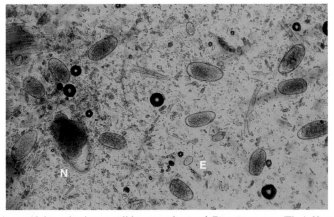

Fig. 1.92. Fecal sample containing mixed strongylid eggs and several *Eimeria* oocysts (E). A *Nematodirus* sp. egg is also present, but slightly out of focus (N).

PARASITE: *Cryptosporidium parvum, C. andersoni* (Figure 1.93)

Taxonomy: Protozoan (coccidia).

Geographic Distribution: Worldwide.

Location in Host: *Cryptosporidium parvum* is an intestinal parasite of ruminants, camelids, and other mammals. *Cryptosporidium andersoni* is a parasite of the bovine abomasum and may also infect camelids.

Life Cycle: Ruminants are infected by ingestion of oocysts. Oocysts are infective as soon as they are passed in the manure and are very resistant to environmental conditions.

Laboratory Diagnosis: Very small oocysts are seen with Sheather's sugar centrifugal flotation exam. Fecal smears can also be stained with acid-fast stains or examined by immunodiagnostic techniques. *Cryptosporidium andersoni* oocysts are slightly larger than those of *C. parvum.*

Size: *C. parvum*   4–5 μm in diameter
          C. andersoni   7 μm × 5 μm

Clinical Importance: Infections with *C. parvum* may be subclinical or cause diarrhea of varying severity in young animals. Some isolates of *C. parvum* can infect both humans and ruminants. *Cryptosporidium andersoni* may cause chronic abomasal infections in cattle, including adults, although it appears to have little economic significance.

PARASITE: *Giardia duodenalis*, **also identified as** *G. lamblia, intestinalis, bovis*, **etc.** (Figures 1.94–1.95, 1.105)

Taxonomy: Protozoan (flagellate). The number of species is currently under revision.

Geographic Distribution: Worldwide.

Location in Host: Small intestine of ruminants and camelids.

Life Cycle: *Giardia* cysts passed in the feces infect other animals when ingested in the environment. Following excystation, trophozoites inhabit the small intestine.

Laboratory Diagnosis: Small cysts can be found in fecal samples using centrifugal flotation procedures (33% $ZnSO_4$ flotation solution preferred). Trichrome-stained fecal smears and immunodiagnostic tests can also be used.

Size: cysts   9–13 × 7–9 μm
          trophozoites   12–17 × 7–10 μm

Clinical Importance: Many animals are infected, particularly when young, but clinical disease is uncommon.

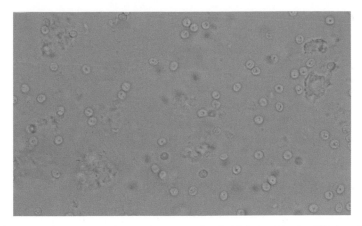

Fig. 1.93. The small oocysts of *Cryptosporidium* are best seen using the high-dry objective (40×) on the microscope. They are highly refractile and often appear to have a single black dot in the center.

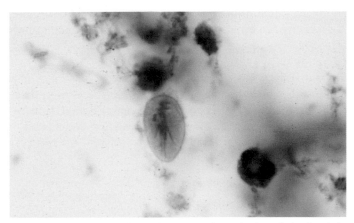

Fig. 1.94. Although small, *Giardia* cysts contain internal structures that make them distinctive. A drop of Lugol's iodine on the slide can help in visualizing internal structure. Photo courtesy of Dr. Robert Ridley, College of Veterinary Medicine, Kansas State University, Manhattan, KS.

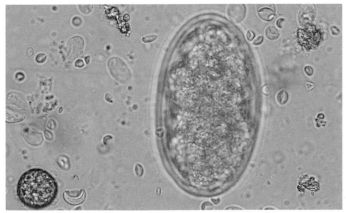

Fig. 1.95. This fecal sample contains *Giardia* sp. cysts, some collapsed (see Fig. 1.34). A strongylid egg is also present in this 40× objective field. Although *Giardia* cysts may be present in large numbers in the feces of ruminants, they are usually not incriminated as a cause of clinical disease.

Helminth Parasites

PARASITE: Strongylid Parasites of Ruminants (Figures 1.95–1.98, 1.92, 1.101, 1.115)

Common name: Various, including brown stomach worm, barber pole worm, hookworm, nodular worm, strongyles, trichostrongyles.

Taxonomy: Nematodes (order Strongylida). Numerous genera belong to this group, including *Ostertagia, Haemonchus, Cooperia, Trichostrongylus, Telodorsagia, Mecistocirrus, Oesophagostomum, Bunostomum, Chabertia, Camelostrongylus,* and *Lamanema.*

Geographic Distribution: Worldwide.

Location in Host: Gastrointestinal tract of ruminant and camelid hosts.

Life Cycle: Adult worms in the gastrointestinal tract produce eggs that develop in manure in the environment. Infective larvae are released onto pasture, where they infect grazing hosts.

Laboratory Diagnosis: Eggs are detected by routine or quantitative fecal flotation procedures. Eggs are similar in appearance and are not easily identified specifically. For diagnosis of genera, culture of feces and identification of infective third-stage larvae are performed. Quantitative egg counts are useful in designing and evaluating parasite control programs.

Size: approx. 65–100 × 34–50 μm, depending on species

Clinical Importance: Virtually all grazing animals are infected with strongylid parasites, and many infections are asymptomatic. Young, nonimmune animals are most susceptible to subclinical and clinical disease, which may include diarrhea, anemia, hypoproteinemia, reduced growth, and death in severe cases. The species of greatest importance vary with host and region.

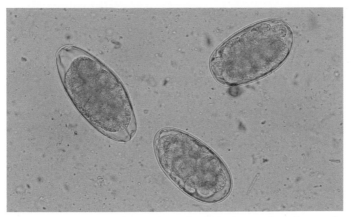

Fig. 1.96. The strongylid egg is the helminth egg seen most often in bovine, small ruminant, and camelid feces. In fresh feces eggs are thin shelled and oval in shape and contain a grapelike cluster of cells (morula). Development to the first larval stage occurs in the egg, and larvated eggs may be seen in older samples. In this sample at least two species are present.

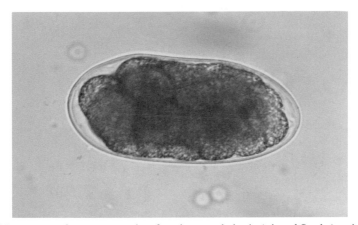

Fig. 1.97. Egg of *Mecistocirrus digitatus,* a parasite of ruminants and pigs in Asia and South America. The parasite produces typical strongylid eggs. Photo courtesy of Dr. Alvin Gajadhar, Centre for Animal Parasitology, CFIA, Saskatoon, Saskatchewan, Canada.

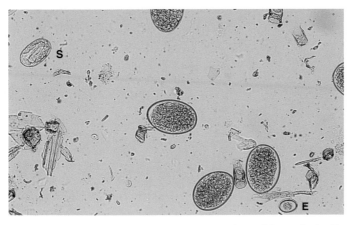

Fig. 1.98. Strongylid eggs in a low-power (10×) field. A smaller, larvated egg of *Strongyloides* (S) and an *Eimeria* oocyst (E) are also present.

77

PARASITE: *Nematodirus* **spp.** (Figures 1.99–1.101, 1.92)
         Common name: Thread-necked worm.

Taxonomy: Nematode (order Strongylida).

Geographic Distribution: Worldwide.

Location in Host: Several species are found in the small intestine of ruminants and camelids.

Life Cycle: Unlike most other strongylids, larvae develop to the infective stage within the egg. Ruminants are infected when they ingest the hatched infective larvae.

Laboratory Diagnosis: Large eggs present in routine or quantitative fecal flotation exams.

  Size: 152–260 × 67–120 µm, depending on species (a similar egg is produced by *Marshallagia marshalli,* a parasite of sheep in the western USA)

Clinical Importance: Most species of *Nematodirus* do not usually cause clinical disease. *Nematodirus battus,* however, is an important cause of lamb diarrhea in some parts of the world.

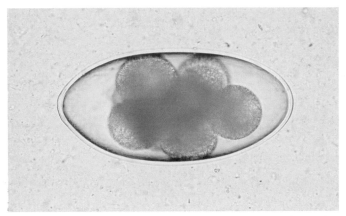

Fig. 1.99. Egg of *Nematodirus* sp. This is one of the few strongylid eggs of ruminants that can be easily identified specifically because of its large size and two to eight distinctive, large cells inside the freshly passed egg. The eggs of *Marshallagia* spp. are similar in size to those of *Nematodirus*. *Marshallagia* spp. are found worldwide but this genus is less common than *Nematodirus*.

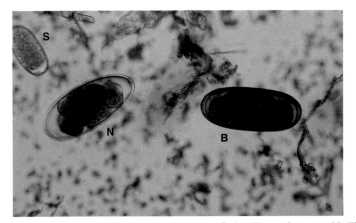

Fig. 1.100. The egg of *Nematodirus battus* (B) is browner than eggs of other *Nematodirus* spp. (N). This sample also contains a typical strongylid egg (S). Photo courtesy of Dr. Gary Zimmerman, Zimmerman Research, Livingston, MT.

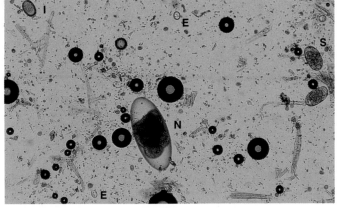

Fig. 1.101. Ovine fecal sample containing strongylid eggs (S), a *Nematodirus* sp. egg (N), an *Eimeria intricata* oocyst (I), and *Eimeria* sp. oocysts (E).

PARASITE: *Trichuris* **spp.** (Figures 1.102, 1.104)
      Common name: Whipworm.

Taxonomy: Nematode (order Enoplida). Several species (*T. ovis, T. discolor*, etc.) occur in ruminants.

Geographic Distribution: Worldwide.

Location in Host: Cecum and colon of ruminants and camelids.

Life Cycle: Eggs produced by adults in the large intestine are passed in the feces. After a minimum of 3 weeks in the environment, eggs reach the infective stage and can infect a host when ingested.

Laboratory Diagnosis: Identification of brown, bipolar-plugged eggs in fecal flotation preparations.

      Size: 70–80 × 30–42 μm

Clinical Importance: Eggs of *Trichuris* are often found in ruminant fecal samples. Clinical disease (diarrhea) is rare and associated with heavy infection.

PARASITE: *Aonchotheca* **(=** *Capillaria***) spp.** (Figures 1.103–1.104)

Taxonomy: Nematode (order Enoplida). These parasites (*A. bovis* in cattle, *A. longipes* in sheep) were formerly included in the genus *Capillaria*. Camelids are also infected with *Aoncotheca*.

Geographic Distribution: Worldwide.

Location in Host: Small intestine of ruminants and camelids.

Life Cycle: Parasite eggs are shed from the host in manure. Infection follows ingestion of infective eggs in the environment.

Laboratory Diagnosis: Eggs with bipolar plugs are detected by fecal flotation procedures. Although they are similar to *Trichuris* (whipworm) eggs, *Aonchotheca* spp. eggs are smaller.

      Size: 45–50 × 22–25 μm

Clinical Importance: *Aonchotheca* infection in ruminants is considered clinically insignificant.

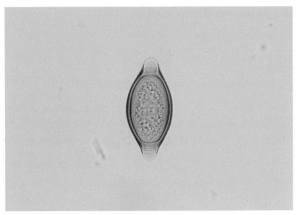

Fig. 1.102. *Trichuris* eggs are common in ruminant feces. They have a thick, brown shell and polar plug at each end.

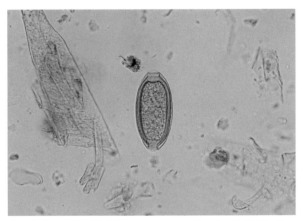

Fig. 1.103. These bipolar *Aonchotheca* (*Capillaria*) eggs can be confused with *Trichuris* eggs but are smaller and less brown in color.

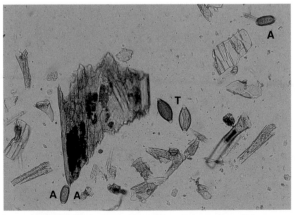

Fig. 1.104. Ruminant fecal sample containing both *Trichuris* (T) and *Aoncotheca* (A) eggs.

Parasite: *Strongyloides papillosus* (Figures 1.105, 1.98)

Taxonomy: Nematode (order Rhabditida).

Geographic Distribution: Worldwide.

Location in Host: Small intestine of ruminants and camelids.

Life Cycle: Eggs shed in the feces hatch, releasing first-stage larvae. After a period of free-living development in the environment, infective third-stage larvae are produced that infect the host by ingestion or penetration of the skin. Transmammary infection also occurs.

Laboratory Diagnosis: Eggs are detected by routine flotation techniques. They are smaller than strongylid eggs and contain a larva when passed in the feces.

Size: 40–60 × 32–40 µm

Clinical Importance: Infection usually has no clinical significance, although very heavy infection may produce severe diarrhea.

Parasite: *Toxocara vitulorum* (Figure 1.106)
Common name: Roundworm.

Taxonomy: Nematode (order Ascaridida).

Geographic Distribution: Worldwide, but rare in cattle in North America.

Location in Host: Small intestine of cattle and bison.

Life Cycle: Cattle are infected following the ingestion of larvated eggs in the environment. Larvae migrate into tissues and form a somatic reservoir that is activated in pregnancy. Egg-producing adult infections occur primarily in calves as a result of transmammary transmission.

Laboratory Diagnosis: Detection of typical ascarid-type eggs with flotation procedures.

Size: 75–95 × 60–75 µm

Clinical Importance: Infection with adult worms occurs in calves less than 6 months of age. Small to moderate infection may be tolerated without signs of disease, but diarrhea, weight loss, and death can occur in heavy infection.

Parasite: *Skrjabinema* spp. (Figure 1.107)
Common name: Pinworm.

Taxonomy: Nematode (Order Oxyurida).

Geographic Distribution: Worldwide.

Location in Host: Cecum of sheep, goats, some wild ruminant species and some camelids.

Life Cycle: Female worms deposit eggs on the perianal skin. Eggs fall off the host, become dispersed in the environment, and are eaten by other animals.

Laboratory Diagnosis: Eggs are rarely seen in routine fecal exams because they are not deposited in the feces.

Size: 47–63 µm × 27–36 µm

Clinical Importance: Clinically insignificant.

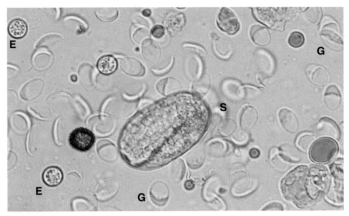

Fig. 1.105. *Strongyloides* eggs may be confused with more common strongylid eggs. The two egg types can be easily distinguished because *Strongyloides* eggs are smaller and contain a fully formed larva when passed in the feces. This calf fecal sample contains a larvated *Strongyloides* egg (S) as well as numerous collapsed *Giardia* cysts (G). Several small *Eimeria* oocysts (E) are also present. Most coccidia spp. oocysts are larger than *Giardia* cysts.

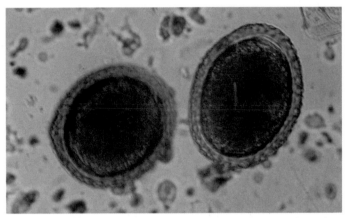

Fig. 1.106. *Toxocara vitulorum* eggs have the thick shell typical of ascarids. *Neoascaris* is rare in cattle in North America. Photo courtesy of Dr. Gil Myers, Myers Parasitological Service, Magnolia, TN, and Dr. Eugene Lyons, Department of Veterinary Science, University of Kentucky, Lexington, KY.

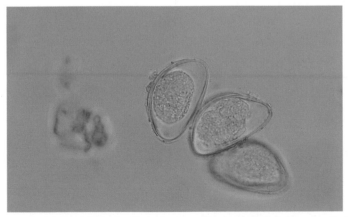

Fig. 1.107. *Skrjabinema*, the ruminant pinworm. Pinworm eggs often appear flattened on one side. These eggs are rarely found in fecal exams because they are not passed in the feces.

Parasite: *Muellerius capillaris, Protostrongylus* spp. (Figures 1.108–1.111)

Taxonomy: Nematodes (order Strongylida).

Geographic Distribution: Worldwide.

Location in Host: Lung parenchyma of sheep, goats, and some deer.

Life Cycle: Infection of small ruminants follows ingestion of infected snail or slug intermediate hosts while grazing. Snails are infected when they eat first-stage larvae in the feces.

Laboratory Diagnosis: The Baermann Test is used for detection of first-stage larvae. *Muellerius* has a kinked tail with an accessory spine, in contrast to the plain tail of *Protostrongylus*.

Size:	*Muellerius*	300–320 μm
	Protostrongylus	340–400 μm

Clinical Importance: Most cases are asymptomatic. Heavy infections may cause clinical disease, especially in goats infected with *Muellerius*.

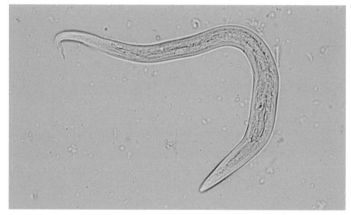

Fig. 1.108. Iodine-stained *Muellerius* larva.

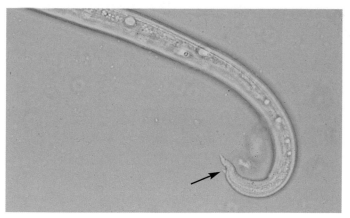

Fig. 1.109. *Muellerius* larvae can be easily identified by the presence of a kinked tail and accessory spine (*arrow*) at the end of the tail.

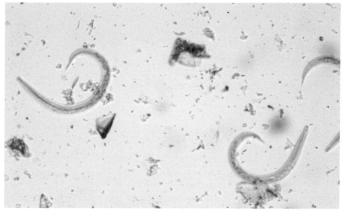

Fig. 1.110. *Protostrongylus* larvae have a plain tail without the kink and accessory spine seen in *Muellerius* larvae. Photo courtesy of Dr. Alvin Gajadhar, Centre for Animal Parasitology, CFIA, Saskatoon, Saskatchewan, Canada.

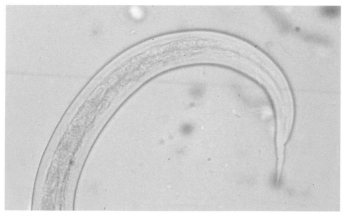

Fig. 1.111. Higher magnification view of the simple tail of a *Protostrongylus* first-stage larva in feces. Photo courtesy of Dr. Alvin Gajadhar, Centre for Animal Parasitology, CFIA, Saskatoon, Saskatchewan, Canada.

PARASITE: *Dictyocaulus* spp. (Figures 1.112–1.113)
        Common name: Lungworm.

Taxonomy: Nematode (order Strongylida). Species include *D. viviparus* (cattle, camelids), *D. filaria* (sheep, goat, camel), *D. cameli* (camel).

Geographic Distribution: Worldwide.

Location in Host: Trachea, bronchi, and bronchioles.

Life Cycle: First-stage larvae are passed in the feces of the host. Infective third-stage larvae develop on pasture and are ingested during grazing. Larvae migrate from the intestine to the respiratory tract and become mature.

Laboratory Diagnosis: The Baermann Test is used to detect first-stage larvae in fresh feces. Some larvated eggs may also be present in fresh feces.

Size: *D. viviparus*   300–360 μm
             D. filaria   550–580 μm

Clinical Importance: Heavy infections may cause severe respiratory signs, especially in cattle. Disease is usually seen in young animals before immunity develops.

PARASITE: *Moniezia* spp. (Figures 1.114–1.116)
        Common name: Tapeworm.

Taxonomy: Cestode. Species include *M. benedeni, M. expansa.*

Geographic Distribution: Worldwide.

Location in Host: Small intestine of ruminants and camelids.

Life Cycle: Tapeworm eggs are shed in segments from the host. Ruminants are infected following ingestion of the intermediate host (free-living pasture mites) containing the tapeworm larvae.

Laboratory Diagnosis: Eggs may be found in fecal flotation tests, but infection is usually recognized when owners see tapeworm segments on the animal or in the environment.

Size: 65–75 μm in diameter

Clinical Importance: In general, little clinical importance, although there are anecdotal reports that heavy infection may cause reduced growth in young animals.

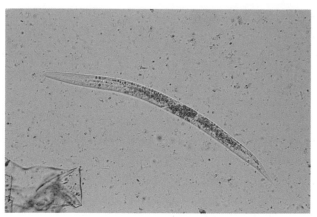

Fig. 1.112. *Dictyocaulus viviparus* first-stage larva. Intestinal cells contain characteristic dark food granules. *Dictyocaulus filaria* larvae have a small knob at the anterior end that is not present in *D. viviparus* larvae.

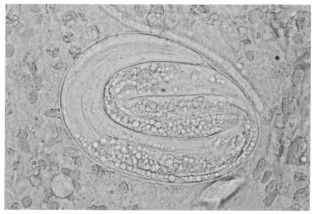

Fig. 1.113. Although *Dictyocaulus* larvae are most often seen in fecal samples, unhatched eggs may also be found in feces and samples collected from the trachea. The dark food granules are evident even in this unhatched *Dictyocaulus* larva. Photo courtesy of Dr. Jeffrey F. Williams, Vanson HaloSource, Inc., Redmond, WA.

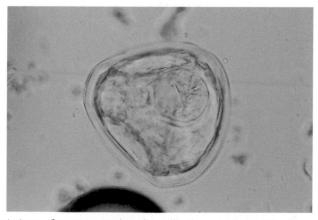

Fig. 1.114. Eggs of *Moniezia* are often square or triangular, unlike the more common round or oval shape of parasite eggs. The presence of the embryo with its six hooks clearly identifies these structures as tapeworm eggs. In this egg, four hooks are visible.

PARASITE: *Thysanosoma, Stilesia* (Figure 1.117)

Taxonomy: Cestodes.

Geographic Distribution: *Stilesia* is found in Europe, Africa, and Asia, while *Thysanosoma* is confined to North and South America. In the USA its distribution appears to be limited to the western states.

Location in Host: Bile ducts of ruminants, especially sheep, and camelids.

Life Cycle: Although these tapeworms have not been extensively studied, it is thought that their intermediate hosts may be oribatid mites. Like *Moniezia,* the definitive host is infected following ingestion of the intermediate host.

Laboratory Diagnosis: Tapeworm segments are passed in the feces and eggs may be found in fecal flotation tests.

Size: approx. 30 × 20 μm

Clinical Importance: These tapeworms have no economic importance unless they are present in large enough numbers to cause liver condemnation.

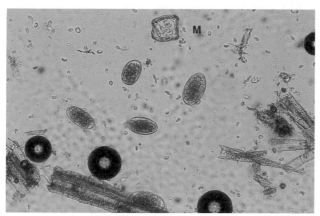

Fig. 1.115. *Moniezia* sp. egg (M) and several ruminant strongylid eggs.

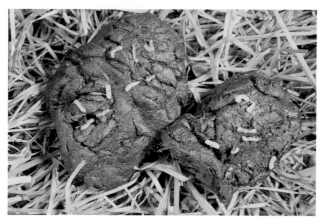

Fig. 1.116. Owners may be alarmed by the presence of *Moniezia* segments in the feces of their animals. Tapeworm segments are seen most often in the manure of young animals. Photo courtesy of Dr. Jeffrey F. Williams, Vanson HaloSource, Inc., Redmond, WA.

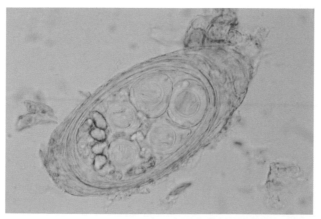

Fig. 1.117. Packet of *Thysanosoma* eggs from a sheep. The eggs lack the pyriform apparatus seen in *Moniezia* eggs. Hooks can easily be seen in the eggs. The entire packet of eggs is 124 × 62 μm. Photo courtesy of Dr. Ellis Greiner, College of Veterinary Medicine, University of Florida, Gainesville, FL.

PARASITE: *Fasciola hepatica* (Figure 1.118)
Common name: Liver fluke.

Taxonomy: Trematode.

Geographic Distribution: Worldwide. A similar species, *F. gigantica,* is also found in Africa, Asia, and Hawaii.

Location in Host: Adults in the bile ducts of cattle, sheep, goats, camelids, and a variety of other animals, including dogs, horses, and humans.

Life Cycle: Miracidia hatch from the eggs and invade an appropriate snail host. Cercariae emerging from the snail encyst on vegetation and are ingested by host animals. Larvae leave the gastrointestinal tract and migrate through the liver to reach the bile ducts.

Laboratory Diagnosis: Large brown eggs are detected using a sedimentation procedure. Eggs may be difficult to detect and not indicative of the level of infection in a herd. A commercially available apparatus, the Flukefinder®, simplifies the sedimentation procedure (see the section "Fecal Sedimentation" above).

Size: 130–150 × 63–90 µm

Clinical Importance: *Fasciola* infections in ruminants may cause significant production losses. Sheep are particularly susceptible and heavy infection may be fatal. Chronically infected animals can develop anemia and unthriftiness.

PARASITE: *Paramphistomum* **spp.** (Figure 1.119)
Common name: Rumen fluke.

Taxonomy: Trematode. Other genera belonging to this family include *Cotylophoron* and *Calicophoron.*

Geographic Distribution: Worldwide.

Location in Host: Adult flukes in the rumen of cattle, sheep, other ruminants, and camelids.

Life Cycle: Eggs passed in the feces of the host animal hatch in water, liberating miracidia, which infect snails. Following development in the snail, cercariae are released, which encyst on vegetation. Definitive hosts are infected by ingesting fluke metacercariae while grazing.

Laboratory Diagnosis: Eggs of paramphistomes are similar to those of *Fasciola*. They are best recovered using a sedimentation procedure, but examination of fecal material will not detect immature flukes, which are the most pathogenic stage of infection.

Size: approx. 114–175 × 65–100 µm, depending on species

Clinical Importance: Clinical disease is rare in North America. In other parts of the world, larval paramphistomes in the duodenum and upper ileum are reported to cause enteritis leading to diarrhea, emaciation, and death in severe cases.

PARASITE: *Dicrocoelium dendriticum* (Figure 1.120)

Taxonomy: Trematode.

Geographic Distribution: Europe, Asia, sporadic occurrence in North America.

Location in Host: Bile ducts of domestic and wild ruminants, pigs, dogs, horses, rabbits.

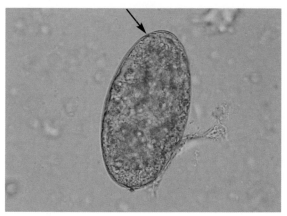

Fig. 1.118. *Fasciola hepatica* egg. These large eggs have an operculum (*arrow*) and look similar to eggs of rumen flukes, although *Paramphistomum* eggs are slightly larger (about 160 μm) and less brown in color.

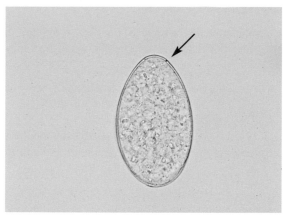

Fig. 1.119. Paramphistome eggs. These eggs will not be detected with routine flotation tests. The operculum of this egg can be seen as a discontinuity in the outline of the eggshell (*arrow*). Photo courtesy of Dr. Robert Ridley, College of Veterinary Medicine, Kansas State University, Manhattan, KS.

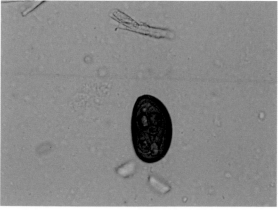

Fig. 1.120. *Dicrocoelium dendriticum* eggs contain a fully formed miracidium, tend to be flattened on one side, and are smaller than eggs of *Fasciola* and the paramphistome flukes.

Life Cycle: Larvae in eggs are ingested by snails. Ants act as the second intermediate host, and the final host is infected while grazing. Larval flukes enter bile ducts directly and do not migrate through the liver.

Laboratory Diagnosis: A sedimentation test will detect the small, brown, operculate eggs in the feces.

   Size: 38–45 μm × 22–30 μm

Clinical Importance: In heavy infections, extensive cirrhosis of the liver can develop, leading to anemia and weight loss.

PARASITE: ***Eurytrema pancreaticum*** (Figure 1.121)

Taxonomy: Trematode.

Geographic Distribution: Asia, parts of South America.

Location in Host: Adult flukes are found in the pancreatic ducts of small ruminants, cattle, camels, pigs, and occasionally humans. Flukes are also occasionally found in the bile ducts and small intestine.

Life Cycle: The eggs produced by adult flukes leave the host in manure. Snails are the first intermediate host. A grasshopper or cricket second intermediate host transmits the infection when ingested by the final host.

Laboratory Diagnosis: A sedimentation test will detect the small, brown eggs in the feces.

   Size: 44–48 × 23–36 μm

Clinical Importance: Many infections are subclinical. Heavy worm burdens can cause fibrosis of the ducts and pancreatic atrophy, resulting in weight loss and poor condition.

PARASITE: ***Schistosoma* spp.** (Figure 1.122)

Taxonomy: Trematode. Several species infect ruminants, camels, horses, and pigs, including *S. bovis, S. mattheei, S. japonicum.*

Geographic Distribution: Africa, Asia.

Location in Host: Most important species are found in the portal mesenteric veins of the host.

Life Cycle: Eggs in host feces hatch in water, releasing the miracidia, which enter the snail intermediate host. Cercariae produced by multiplication within the snail are released and penetrate the skin of the definitive host. There is no second intermediate host in the life cycle.

Laboratory Diagnosis: A saline sedimentation procedure is used to detect eggs in manure. Fecal examination is most useful in early infection because egg production declines as infection progresses. Eggs do not have an operculum and most are spindle shaped. In some species a spine is present on one end of the egg.

   Size: 130–280 × 38–85 μm, depending on species

Clinical Importance: Disease results from the host reaction to the presence of parasite eggs in tissue. Clinical signs may occur in heavy infections, including diarrhea, anemia, and wasting.

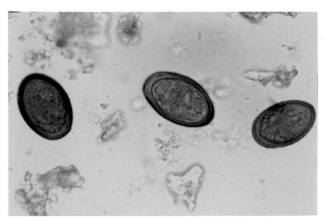

Fig. 1.121. The eggs of *Eurytrema* are similar in appearance to those of *Dicrocoelium*. Photo courtesy of Dr. Alvin Gajadhar, Centre for Animal Parasitology, CFIA, Saskatoon, Saskatchewan, Canada.

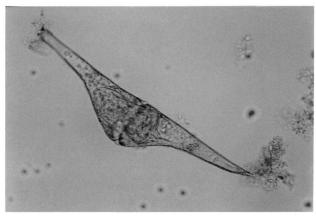

Fig. 1.122. Ruminant schistosomes typically produce a spindle-shaped egg. This egg of *Schistosoma spindale*, an Asian species, has a spine at one end. Photo courtesy of Dr. Alvin Gajadhar, Centre for Animal Parasitology, CFIA, Saskatoon, Saskatchewan, Canada.

Horses

In comparison to dogs and cats and ruminants, the diversity of parasite eggs and oocysts frequently encountered in equine feces is much reduced. The most common finding in equine samples is the strongylid egg. Horses are infected with 54 strongylid species, although individual species cannot be determined. The parasites shown in this section can also infect other equid species. Parasites illustrated in other sections may not be extensively covered here and references are given to figures elsewhere in the book.

Helminth Ova and Protozoan Cysts
as found in freshly voided feces of
Horses

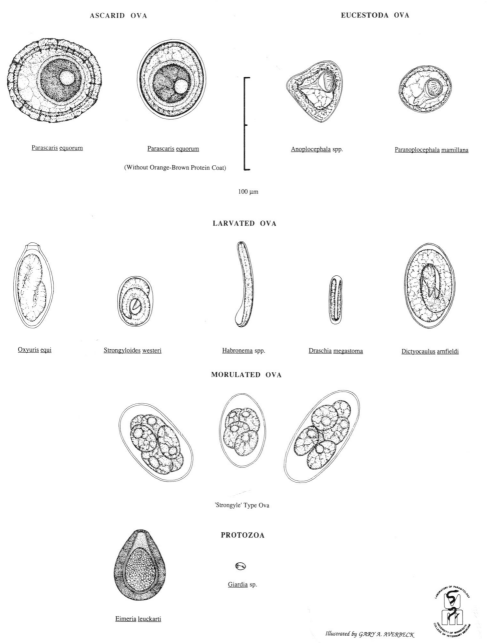

ASCARID OVA

EUCESTODA OVA

Parascaris equorum

Parascaris equorum

(Without Orange-Brown Protein Coat)

100 μm

Anoplocephala spp.

Paranoplocephala mamillana

LARVATED OVA

Oxyuris equi

Strongyloides westeri

Habronema spp.

Draschia megastoma

Dictyocaulus arnfieldi

MORULATED OVA

'Strongyle' Type Ova

PROTOZOA

Giardia sp.

Eimeria leuckarti

Illustrated by GARY A. AVERBECK

Fig. 1.123. Common parasites found in fecal samples of horses. Fig. courtesy of Dr. Bert Stromberg and Mr. Gary Averbeck, College of Veterinary Medicine, University of Minnesota, Minneapolis, MN.

95

Protozoan Parasites

PARASITE: *Eimeria leuckarti* (Figure 1.124)

Taxonomy: Protozoan (coccidia).

Geographic Distribution: Worldwide.

Location in Host: Small intestine of horses and donkeys.

Life Cycle: Oocysts leave the host in the manure. Sporulation occurs in the environment, and new hosts are infected by ingestion of infective oocysts.

Laboratory Diagnosis: Infection is diagnosed by finding the large, deep brown oocysts in the feces. A sedimentation procedure has been recommended, but oocysts can also be seen with flotation procedures.

Size: 80–88 × 55–59 μm

Clinical Importance: Infection appears to have little clinical significance in horses, although rare cases of diarrhea have been reported. Infections are seen only in young animals.

PARASITE: *Giardia duodenalis, Cryptosporidium parvum* (Figures 1.125–1.126, 1.29, 1.32–1.38, 1.93–1.94)

Taxonomy: Protozoa (*Giardia,* flagellates*; Cryptosporidium,* coccidia).

Geographic Location: Worldwide.

Location in Host: Small intestine.

Laboratory Diagnosis: As in other hosts, *Giardia* cysts can be detected with 33% $ZnSO_4$ centrifugal flotation, and *Cryptosporidium* oocysts with Sheather's sugar centrifugal flotation. Both organisms can also be found in fecal smears with appropriate stains and by non-host-specific immunodiagnostic tests.

Clinical Importance: Both infections occur most frequently in young animals but are rarely associated with clinical disease.

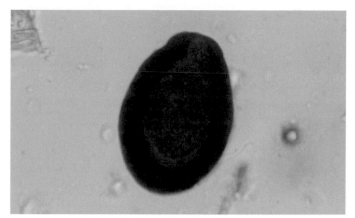

Fig. 1.124. The large size and deep brown color of the oocysts of *Eimeria leuckarti* make them very distinctive. They are seen in feces of young horses.

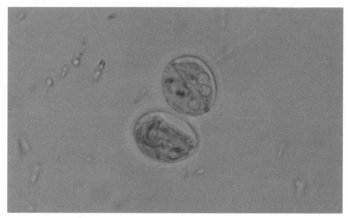

Fig. 1.125. Fecal flotation tests containing iodine-stained *Giardia* cysts.

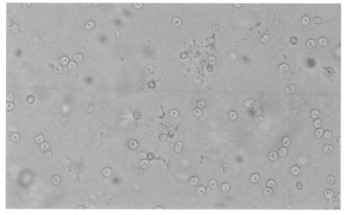

Fig. 1.126. *Cryptosporidium* oocysts in a sugar flotation preparation.

Helminth Parasites

PARASITE: **Equine Strongylid Parasites** (Figures 1.127–1.129, 1.132, 1.139)
        Common name: Various, including bloodworm, small and large strongyle.

Taxonomy: Nematodes (order Strongylida). Numerous genera belong to this group, including the large strongyles (*Strongylus vulgaris*, etc.), the small strongyles (cyathostomes), and *Trichostrongylus axei*.

Geographic Distribution: Worldwide.

Location in Host: Cecum and colon (with the exception of *T. axei*, a parasite of the stomach).

Life Cycle: Eggs released by adult worms in the large bowel develop in feces in the environment. Infective larvae on pasture are ingested by grazing horses. Large and small strongyles undergo a period of development in the intestinal wall (small strongyles) or in extra-intestinal tissue (large strongyles) before maturing in the bowel lumen.

Laboratory Diagnosis: Eggs are detected on routine fecal flotation. Eggs are similar in appearance and are not routinely identified specifically. Quantitative egg counts are useful in designing parasite control programs.

   Size: variable, with considerable overlap among species; eggs approx. 60–120 × 35–60 μm

Clinical Importance: Virtually all grazing horses are infected with strongylid parasites. Many low to moderate infections are subclinical, although they may cause reduced weight gain and performance. Young, nonimmune animals are most susceptible to clinical disease, which may include diarrhea, colic, and hypoproteinemia.

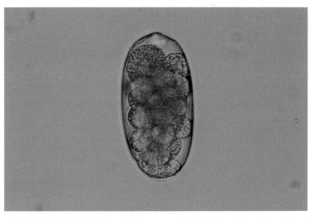

Fig. 1.127. Equine strongylid eggs in fresh fecal samples are typical of the order, with a thin shell surrounding a central group of cells. In warm weather, larvae may form within 1–2 days.

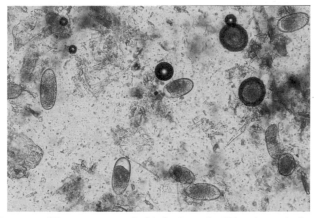

Fig. 1.128. Several equine strongylid eggs are present in this fecal sample. Although egg size is variable, there is too much overlap for size to be a useful characteristic for identification of individual species. Two *Parascaris* (roundworm) eggs are also present.

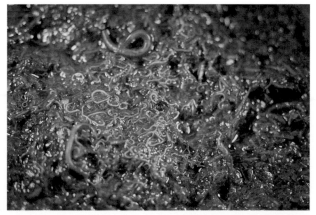

Fig. 1.129. Large and small equine strongyles in bowel contents. These parasites are sometimes present in the manure of horses, particularly in cases of larval cyathostomiasis. Manure of horses with this condition may contain large numbers of larval small strongyles less than an inch in length. Photo courtesy of Dr. Jeffrey F. Williams, Vanson HaloSource, Inc., Redmond, WA.

PARASITE: *Parascaris equorum* (Figures 1.130–1.132, 1.128)
Common name: Roundworm.

Taxonomy: Nematode (order Ascaridida).

Geographic Distribution: Worldwide.

Location in Host: Small intestine of horses and other equids.

Life Cycle: Infective larvae develop in eggs passed in the feces of horses. Infection occurs by ingestion of larvated eggs. Larvae migrate through the liver and lungs of the host before returning to the small intestine to mature.

Laboratory Diagnosis: Flotation procedures will detect the typical thick-shelled ascarid eggs.

Size: 90–100 μm in diameter

Following treatment with some anthelmintics, adult ascarids may be passed in manure. These worms will be much larger than any other equine helminths, with females reaching 50 cm in length.

Clinical Importance: Adult worms are common in young horses, infrequent in adults. Heavy infections can cause respiratory signs (from migrating larvae), ill-thrift, colic, diarrhea, and intestinal obstruction that may be fatal.

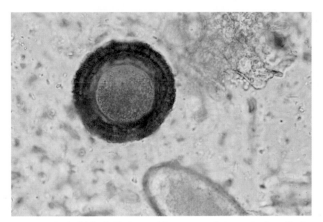

Fig. 1.130. *Parascaris* eggs are typical, thick-shelled ascarid eggs containing a single cell when passed in the feces. Fig. 1.128 shows *Parascaris* eggs at a lower magnification.

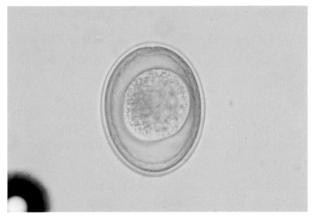

Fig. 1.131. *Parascaris* eggs may lose the rough, proteinaceous coat on the eggshell, but they can still be identified as ascarid eggs by the thick shell and single cell inside the egg.

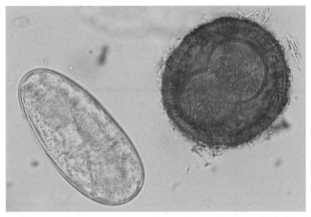

Fig. 1.132. Larvated strongylid egg and *Parascaris* egg that has undergone the first cell division. The fecal sample containing these eggs was fresh when collected but was not examined for some time, allowing development to occur.

PARASITE: *Strongyloides westeri* (Figures 1.133, 1.98)
Common name: Threadworm.

Taxonomy: Nematode (order Rhabditida).

Geographic Distribution: Worldwide.

Location in Host: Small intestine.

Life Cycle: Patent infections develop primarily by transmammary infection of foals. Larvated eggs passed in the feces of foals lead to the development of infective larvae that can penetrate skin or be ingested. In adult horses, larvae migrate to tissues and form a somatic larval reservoir.

Laboratory Diagnosis: Small, larvated eggs are detected by flotation procedures.

Size: 40–52 × 32–40 μm

Clinical Importance: Clinical disease occurs only in foals. Heavy burdens can produce severe diarrhea and dehydration. Respiratory signs may develop associated with larval migration.

PARASITE: *Oxyuris equi* (Figures 1.134–1.135)
Common name: Pinworm.

Taxonomy: Nematode (order Oxyurida). *Probstmayria vivipara* is a less common pinworm of horses.

Geographic Distribution: Worldwide.

Location in Host: Large intestine of horses and other equids.

Life Cycle: Horses ingest infective eggs. Adult female worms migrate to the perianal region and lay clusters of sticky eggs. These eventually are rubbed off the horse and contaminate the environment.

Laboratory Diagnosis: Because eggs are attached to hairs in the perianal region, they are not often seen in flotation tests. A more successful procedure for recovering eggs is the "Scotch tape test." A piece of clear adhesive tape is touched to the skin in the perianal area and then taped onto a microscope slide and examined. Pinworm eggs can easily be seen through the tape.

Size: 85–95 × 40–45 μm

Clinical Importance: Egg-laying activities of the female worms produce intense pruritus. Horses bite at and rub the perineal region, leading to a "rat-tailed" appearance and possible secondary trauma.

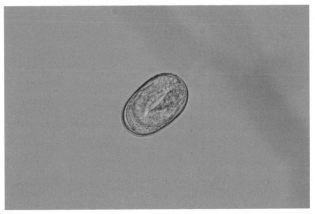

Fig. 1.133. Egg of *Strongyloides westeri,* the horse threadworm. These eggs are usually seen only in the feces of young horses. *Strongyloides* eggs are already larvated when passed in the feces, and they are smaller than strongylid eggs. Fig. 1.98 shows both *Strongyloides* and strongylid eggs of ruminants, which have a similar size relationship to equine species.

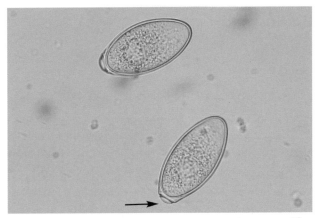

Fig. 1.134. *Oxyuris* eggs are asymmetrical with a polar plug (*arrow*). Eggs embryonate rapidly and are usually seen with a larva inside.

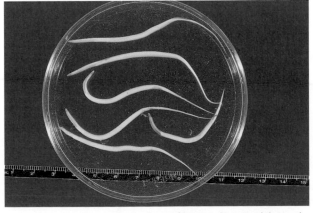

Fig. 1.135. Adult pinworms are occasionally seen in the feces of horses. *Oxyuris* adults reach a maximum size of 15 cm and can be recognized by their thin, pointed tails. Photo courtesy of Dr. Jeffrey F. Williams, Vanson HaloSource, Inc., Redmond, WA.

PARASITE: *Habronema* spp., *Draschia megastoma* (Figure 1.136)

Taxonomy: Nematodes (order Spirurida).

Geographic Distribution: Worldwide.

Location in Host: Stomach of horses and donkeys.

Life Cycle: Adult worms are found in tumor-like masses in the stomach. Larvated eggs are passed in the feces and are ingested by fly larvae intermediate hosts. Infective worm larvae deposited by adult flies around the lips of horses make their way into the mouth and to the stomach.

Laboratory Diagnosis: The larvated eggs passed in the feces are too dense to float in most flotation solutions. A sedimentation procedure is recommended for detection.

Clinical Importance: Gastritis resulting in poor growth may develop. If flies deposit third-stage larvae on a wound, a condition known as "summer sore" can occur, in which larvae survive and prevent wound healing. Since the introduction of macrolide anthelmintics, infection with these species has become much less common.

PARASITE: *Dictyocaulus arnfeldi* (Figure 1.137)
Common name: Lungworm.

Taxonomy: Nematode (order Strongylida).

Geographic Distribution: Worldwide.

Location in Host: Bronchi and bronchioles of horses and donkeys.

Life Cycle: Adult worms in the respiratory tract produce larvated eggs that hatch before or soon after leaving the host. Eggs and/or larvae are coughed up, swallowed, and passed in the feces. Larvae develop to the infective third stage in the environment and are ingested by grazing horses.

Laboratory Diagnosis: Larvated eggs may be detected in feces with flotation tests. However, eggs hatch rapidly or even before leaving the host, so a Baermann Test for the first-stage larvae is the preferred technique for diagnosis. While lungworms readily mature in donkeys, they may not mature in horses, making diagnosis more difficult.

Size:	eggs	74–96 × 46–58 μm
	larvae	420–480 μm

Clinical Importance: Bronchitis and pneumonia may develop. Infections appear to be tolerated better by donkeys than by horses.

PARASITE: *Anoplocephala perfoliata, A. magna,* and *Paranoplocephala mamillana* (Figures 1.138–1.139)
Common name: Tapeworm.

Taxonomy: Cestodes.

Geographic Distribution: Worldwide.

Location in Host: Small intestine of horses and donkeys.

Life Cycle: Eggs passed in the feces are ingested by free-living pasture mites. Horses are infected during grazing when they ingest mites containing tapeworm cysticercoid larvae.

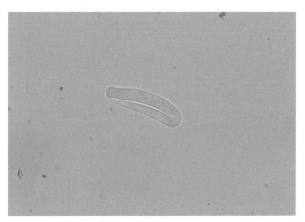

Fig. 1.136. This *Habronema* larva was teased from the uterus of an adult female worm. It will appear in a fecal exam in this form surrounded by a very thin shell.

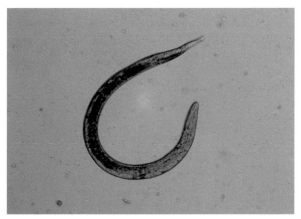

Fig. 1.137. The only parasitic nematode larvae that would be expected in the fresh feces of horses are those of *Dictyocaulus*. The large larva has a small spike at the end of the tail. See also Fig. 1.113 for *Dictyocaulus* eggs that may be seen in tracheal fluid samples. Photo courtesy of Dr. Craig Reinemeyer, East Tennessee Clinical Research, Knoxville, TN.

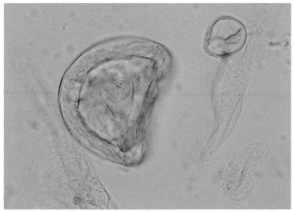

Fig. 1.138. The egg of the equine tapeworm *Anoplocephala* is similar in appearance to that of the ruminant tapeworm *Moniezia*. The eggs of both genera are often irregularly shaped. A pyriform apparatus surrounds the embryo, which has six hooks (hexacanth).

Laboratory Diagnosis: Flotation procedures for detection of eggs in fecal samples are used, but false-negative results are common.

	Size:	
	A. perfoliata	65–80 μm in diameter
	other species	50–60 μm

Clinical Importance: Most tapeworm infections are asymptomatic. Disease has been associated with *A. perfoliata*. These parasites cluster at the ileo-cecal junction, where heavy infection can cause ulceration leading to perforation or intussusception.

Horses may also be infected with some of the trematode (fluke) parasites that affect ruminants. For information on these parasites, see above.

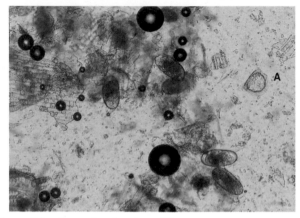

Fig. 1.139. *Anoplocephala* egg (A) and several equine strongylid eggs.

Helminth Ova and Protozoan Cysts
as found in freshly voided feces of
Pigs

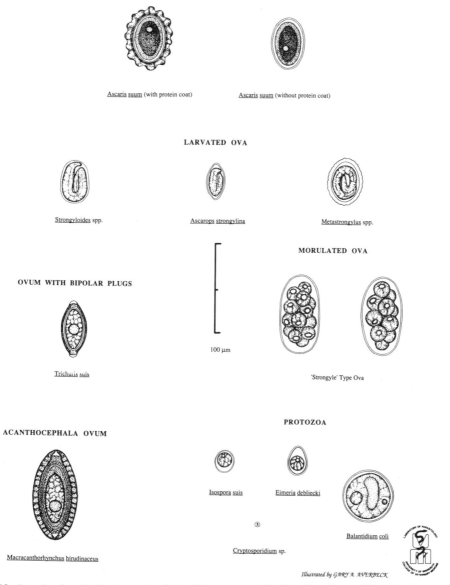

ASCARID OVA

Ascaris suum (with protein coat)   Ascaris suum (without protein coat)

LARVATED OVA

Strongyloides spp.   Ascarops strongylina   Metastrongylus spp.

OVUM WITH BIPOLAR PLUGS

MORULATED OVA

100 μm

Trichuris suis

'Strongyle' Type Ova

ACANTHOCEPHALA OVUM

PROTOZOA

Isospora suis   Eimeria debliecki

Balantidium coli

Macracanthorhynchus hirudinaceus

Cryptosporidium sp.

Illustrated by GARY A. AVERBECK

Fig. 1.140. Parasites found in fecal samples of pigs. Fig. courtesy of Dr. Bert Stromberg and Mr. Gary Averbeck, College of Veterinary Medicine, University of Minnesota, Minneapolis, MN.

Protozoan Parasites

PARASITE: *Eimeria* **spp.,** *Isospora suis* (Figure 1.141)
        Common name: Coccidia.

Taxonomy: Protozoa (coccidia). Eight species of porcine *Eimeria* have been described, including *E. scabra, E. deblieki, E. spinosa.*

Geographic Distribution: Worldwide.

Location in Host: Intestinal tract, location depends on species and stage of development.

Life Cycle: Oocysts are shed in the feces and sporulate rapidly in warm weather. Pigs are infected when they ingest sporulated (infective) oocysts. Transmission of *Isospora suis* is concentrated in the neonatal period of pigs.

Laboratory Diagnosis: *Eimeria* oocysts are detected in feces with flotation procedures. *Isospora suis* oocysts are shed at such a low rate in asymptomatic carriers that detection is very difficult. In clinically affected neonatal pigs, disease usually develops before oocysts are shed, and intestinal mucosal impression smears at necropsy are more effective for diagnosis.

  Size: oocysts vary with species, with a range of 11–35 × 9–20 µm

Clinical Importance: *Eimeria* spp. infections are common in swine but rarely produce clinical disease. In contrast, *Isospora suis* can produce neonatal diarrhea in pigs (5–10 days of age) that may be severe and cause death.

  Swine may also be infected with *Cryptosporidium parvum* and *Giardia intestinalis*. These two protozoan parasites appear to have little clinical significance but are of zoonotic importance. For further information, see listings above.

PARASITE: *Balantidium coli* (Figures 1.142–1.143)

Taxonomy: Protozoan (ciliate).

Geographic Distribution: Worldwide.

Location in Host: Large intestine of swine. May also occasionally infect humans and other primates, camels, dogs, and other animals.

Life Cycle: Infection follows ingestion of cysts shed into the environment from infected swine. The only other stage of the life cycle is the motile trophozoite in the intestinal tract.

Laboratory Diagnosis: Motile trophozoites can be seen in direct fecal smears. Flotation tests are more sensitive for detecting cysts. The kidney-bean-shaped macronucleus is a distinctive feature.

  Size: trophozoites   50–150 µm
             cysts   40–60 µm

Clinical Importance: *Balantidium* is generally asymptomatic in swine, although bloody diarrhea may occur in some hosts.

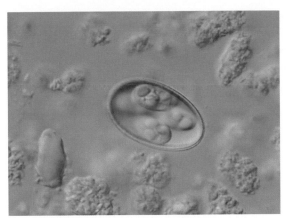

Fig. 1.141. *Eimeria* spp. are the most common coccidia seen in porcine fecal samples. Although several species can infect pigs, they are of little economic importance. Shown here is a sporulated oocyst of *E. scabra*. Photo courtesy of Dr. David Lindsay, Virginia-Maryland Regional College of Veterinary Medicine, Virginia Tech, Blacksburg, VA.

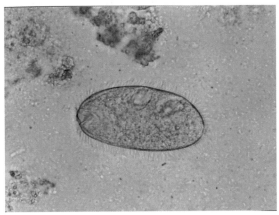

Fig. 1.142. *Balantidium coli* trophozoite in a direct smear. The cilia covering trophozoites can be seen as a halo surrounding the organism. Trophozoites are usually destroyed by fecal flotation procedures. Photo courtesy of Dr. Alvin Gajadhar, Centre for Animal Parasitology, CFIA, Saskatoon, Saskatchewan, Canada.

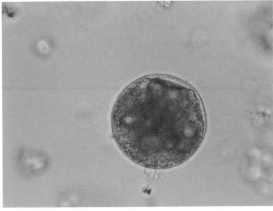

Fig. 1.143. The characteristic kidney-bean-shaped macronucleus of *Balantidium* is faintly visible in this cyst in a porcine fecal sample. The macronucleus is usually easily seen in stained specimens. Photo courtesy of Dr. Alvin Gajadhar, Centre for Animal Parasitology, CFIA, Saskatoon, Saskatchewan, Canada.

Helminth Parasites

PARASITE: *Ascaris suum* (Figure 1.144)
  Common name: Roundworm.

Taxonomy: Nematode (order Ascaridida).

Geographic Distribution: Worldwide.

Location in Host: Small intestine.

Life Cycle: Pigs are infected when they ingest infective eggs in the environment. Following migration through the liver and lungs, adults develop in the small intestine. Like other ascarids, *Ascaris suum* has very resistant eggs that can survive for years in the environment.

Laboratory Diagnosis: Eggs can be detected in feces with routine flotation procedures.

Clinical Importance: *Ascaris suum* is a common and important parasite of swine, even in confinement systems. Larval migration through liver and lung may cause liver condemnation and predispose pigs to bacterial or viral pneumonia. Adult worms in the small intestine may cause reduced growth. Larvae can also migrate and cause disease in other animals and humans.

PARASITE: *Hyostrongylus rubidus*, *Oesophagostomum* **spp.** (Figure 1.145)
  Common name: Red stomach worm (*Hyostrongylus*), nodular worm (*Oesophagostomum*).

Taxonomy: Nematodes (order Strongylida).

Geographic Distribution: Worldwide.

Location in Host: Stomach (*Hyostrongylus)* and large intestine (*Oesophagostomum*) of wild and domestic swine.

Life Cycle: These parasites have a direct life cycle; eggs are shed in the feces and hatch in the environment. Swine are infected following ingestion of third-stage larvae.

Laboratory Diagnosis: Typical strongylid eggs are detected in fecal samples by flotation techniques. Eggs of *Hyostrongylus* and *Oesophagostomum* cannot be distinguished from each other or from less common strongylid parasites of swine, including *Trichostrongylus axei* and *Globocephalus*.

  Size: 69–85 × 39–45 µm

Clinical Importance: These parasites are common in pastured swine. *Hyostrongylus* may cause ulcerative gastritis, resulting in anemia and reduced production. Host response to *Oesophagostomum* larvae in the wall of the intestinal tract leads to the development of nodules that, in heavy infections, can lead to enteritis and reduced production.

PARASITE: *Trichuris suis* (Figure 1.146)
  Common name: Whipworm.

Taxonomy: Nematode (order Enoplida).

Geographic Distribution: Worldwide.

Location in Host: Large intestine of wild and domestic pigs.

Life Cycle: *Trichuris* spp. have a direct life cycle. Pigs are infected following ingestion of infective eggs in the environment. Eggs leave the host in manure and are able to survive for long periods in the environment.

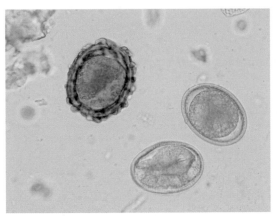

Fig. 1.144. Like other ascarid eggs, those of *Ascaris suum* contain a single cell surrounded by a thick shell when first passed in the feces. In some cases, the rough, brown outer layer of the shell may be absent, as seen in two of the eggs in this figure. *Ascaris suum* eggs are very similar in appearance to those of the human ascarid, *A. lumbricoides*.

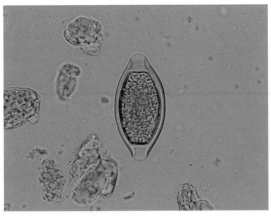

Fig. 1.145. *Hyostrongylus* and *Oesophagostomum* are the most common and important strongylid parasites of swine and produce indistinguishable eggs typical of this group of nematodes. Fecal culture and identification of third-stage larvae are necessary to identify parasite genus.

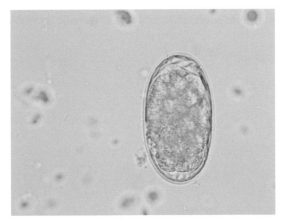

Fig. 1.146. Like other members of the genus, eggs of *Trichuris suis*, the swine whipworm, are football shaped with a polar plug at each end.

Laboratory Diagnosis: Eggs can be detected in routine fecal flotation tests.

Size: 50–60 × 21–25 µm

Clinical Importance: This common helminth infection of swine may cause severe diarrhea and dehydration. Severe infections can produce bloody diarrhea.

PARASITE: *Strongyloides ransomi* (Figures 1.147–1.148, 1.98)
Common name: Threadworm.

Taxonomy: Nematode (order Rhabditida).

Geographic Distribution: Worldwide.

Location in Host: Small intestine.

Life Cycle: Larvated eggs are passed in the feces and hatch in the environment. After a free-living period in the environment, third-stage larvae are produced that infect pigs either through ingestion or skin penetration. Sows carrying larvae in the tissues transmit the parasite through the milk to their litters.

Laboratory Diagnosis: Eggs are detected in fecal samples using flotation techniques. The thin-shelled egg contains a larva in fresh fecal samples.

Size: 40–50 × 20–35 µm

Clinical Importance: *Strongyloides* causes diarrhea in pigs as young as 10 days of age. Severe infections may be fatal.

PARASITE: *Metastrongylus* **spp.** (Figure 1.149)
Common name: Lungworm.

Taxonomy: Nematode (order Strongylida). Several species similar in life cycle and pathogenicity have been described.

Geographic Distribution: Worldwide.

Location in Host: Bronchi and bronchioles of domestic and wild pigs.

Life Cycle: Eggs containing a larva are passed in the feces of pigs. When earthworm intermediate hosts ingest the eggs, they hatch and develop to infective larvae. Swine are infected by ingestion of earthworms containing third-stage larvae.

Laboratory Diagnosis: Larvated eggs are detected in feces by flotation procedures.

Size: 51–63 µm × 33–42 µm

Clinical Importance: These parasites are uncommon in intensively raised swine. Heavy infections, especially in young pigs, can cause clinical respiratory disease.

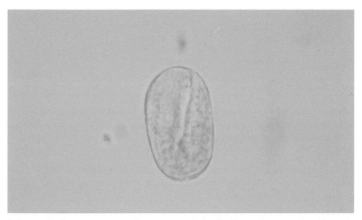

Fig. 1.147. Larvated *Strongyloides* eggs are usually present only in the feces of young pigs. Photo courtesy of Merial.

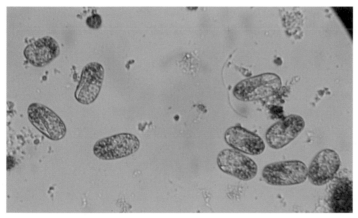

Fig. 1.148. The *Strongyloides* eggs pictured here could be confused with strongylid eggs, but strongylid eggs are larger and do not contain a larva in fresh fecal samples. Fig. 1.98 shows the similar size relationship of ruminant strongylid and *Strongyloides* eggs. Photo courtesy of Dr. T. Bonner Stewart, School of Veterinary Medicine, Louisiana State University, Baton Rouge, LA.

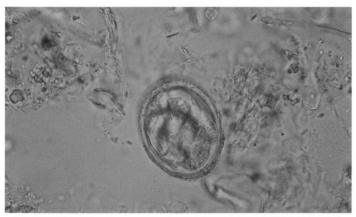

Fig. 1.149. In fresh fecal samples *Metastrongylus* eggs contain a larva and must be differentiated from other larvated parasite eggs found in swine manure.

PARASITE: *Physocephalus sexalatus, Ascarops strongylina* (Figures 1.150–1.151)

Taxonomy: Nematoda (order Spirurida).

Geographic Distribution: Worldwide.

Location in Host: Stomach of domestic and wild pigs.

Life Cycle: Eggs containing larvae are passed in the feces, where they are ingested by beetle intermediate hosts. Pigs are infected following ingestion of larvae in the intermediate host.

Laboratory Diagnosis: A sedimentation procedure is recommended for detecting spirurid parasite eggs. The ellipsoidal eggs of both species are indistinguishable and are larvated when passed in the feces.

Size: 39–45 × 17–26 μm

Clinical Importance: Spirurid parasites are uncommon in intensively raised swine. Most infections are asymptomatic, but heavy infections may produce gastritis, leading to weight loss or failure to gain.

PARASITE: *Fasciola* **spp.,** *Eurytrema pancreaticum, Dicrocoelium dentriticum, Schistosoma* **spp.** (Figure 1.152, 1.113–1.117)

Although swine are not considered to be the primary host for most trematodes, pigs may be infected with trematode parasites (*Fasciola* spp., *Eurytrema pancreaticum, Dicrocoelium dentriticum, Schistosoma* spp.) that also infect ruminants; see Figures 1.118, 1.120–1 and the listings above. Trematode infections of domestic swine would only be seen in pastured pigs because the complicated life cycle of flukes make transmission impossible in confinement operations.

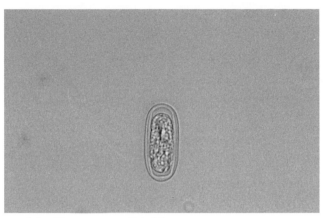

Fig. 1.150. Egg of *Physocephalus*. Photo courtesy of Merial.

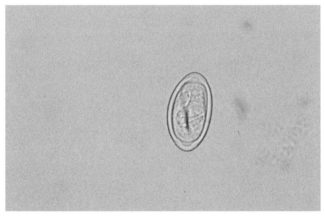

Fig. 1.151. *Ascarops* egg. Spirurid eggs are unlikely to be seen if standard flotation procedures are used. Their larvated eggs have a thick shell (easily appreciated in the *Physocephalus* egg), unlike the thin-shelled eggs of *Strongyloides* or *Metastrongylus*. Photo courtesy of Merial.

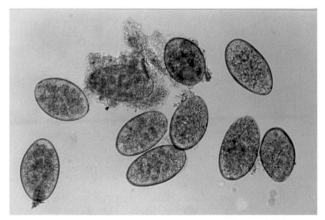

Fig. 1.152. *Fasciola* eggs. Trematode infections are rarely encountered in swine in North America, but are more common in other parts of the world where pigs range freely and infections also occur in other domestic animals. Photo courtesy of Dr. Alvin Gajadhar, Centre for Animal Parasitology, CFIA, Saskatoon, Saskatchewan, Canada.

PARASITE: *Macracanthorhynchus hirudinaceus* (Figure 1.153)
Common name: Thorny-headed worm.

Taxonomy: Acanthocephalan.

Geographic Distribution: Worldwide.

Location in Host: Small intestine.

Life Cycle: Parasite eggs are passed in manure and ingested by beetle intermediate hosts. Swine are infected when they ingest infective larvae (cystacanths) in beetles.

Laboratory Diagnosis: Eggs are not consistently recovered by flotation procedures. A sedimentation procedure should also be performed.

Size: variable, 67–110 × 40–65 μm

Clinical Importance: Acanthocephalan parasites have a proboscis covered with hooks. Attachment of the proboscis causes damage to the intestinal wall. Clinical signs range from none to diarrhea and weight loss. *Macracanthorhynchus* is unlikely to be present in total-confinement systems.

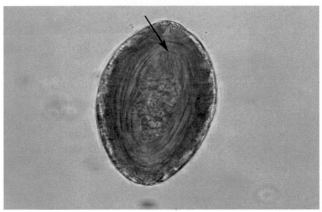

Fig. 1.153. *Macracanthorhynchus hirudinaceus* egg. The embryo (acanthor) is surrounded by several membranes and contains hooks at one end that are often visible (*arrow*). Common tapeworm eggs also contain hooks, but thorny headed worm eggs have a more complex membranous structure and an elongated embryo. Photo courtesy of Dr. Alvin Gajadhar, Centre for Animal Parasitology, CFIA, Saskatoon, Saskatchewan, Canada.

Birds

Protozoan Parasites

PARASITE: *Eimeria* **spp.,** *Isospora* **spp.** (Figures 1.154–1.158, 1.162, 1.164, 1.166, 1.169, 1.174) Common name: Coccidia.

Taxonomy: Protozoa (coccidia). *Eimeria* spp. are common in poultry and other Galliformes and Columbriformes. *Isospora* coccidia species are more common in Passeriformes, Psittaciformes, and Piciformes. Species of coccidia are host specific. *Caryospora, Sarcocystis*, and *Atoxoplasma* are other coccidian genera that infect some birds.

Geographic Distribution: Worldwide.

Location in Host: Primarily in the gastrointestinal tract.

Life Cycle: These parasites have a typical coccidian life cycle. Birds ingest infective oocysts from the environment. Sexual and asexual multiplication occurs within cells of the intestinal tract (some more unusual species are found in other organs). Development culminates in the production of oocysts, which are passed in the feces.

Laboratory Diagnosis: *Eimeria* oocysts are detected with routine flotation procedures. Sporulation of oocysts may be required for species identification.

Size: approx. 10–45 μm in length (oocysts), depending on species

Clinical Importance: Coccidia are common parasites of domestic and wild birds. Many infections are asymptomatic, but under some circumstances coccidia may cause severe diarrhea and death. *Eimeria* spp. are among the most important pathogens in modern poultry-confinement operations.

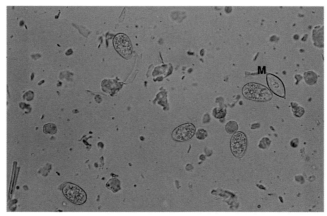

Fig. 1.154. *Eimeria* spp. oocysts from a duck. *Eimeria* species are common parasites of wild and domestic birds. Also present is *Monocystis* (M), a parasite of earthworms.

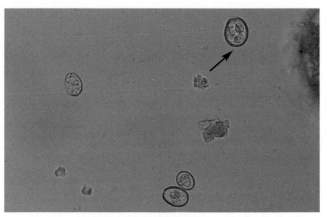

Fig. 1.155. After reaching the environment, *Eimeria* oocysts sporulate; the length of time required for this process is determined by temperature but may take only a few days. This field shows several unsporulated oocysts and one that has sporulated (*arrow*) to contain four sporocysts (three are visible). Sporulated *Isospora* oocysts contain two sporocysts.

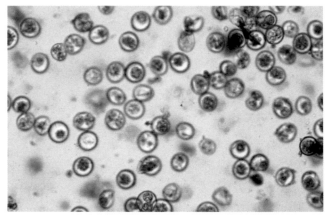

Fig. 1.156. *Isospora* spp. can also be found in birds, as seen in this fecal sample from a crow. Sporulated *Isospora* spp. oocysts contain two sporocysts. Photo courtesy of Dr. Alvin Gajadhar, Centre for Animal Parasitology, CFIA, Saskatoon, Saskatchewan, Canada.

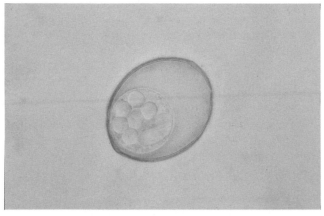

Fig. 1.157. *Caryospora* oocyst. The sporulated oocyst of this genus contains a single sporocyst with eight sporozoites. Photo courtesy of Dr. David Baker, School of Veterinary Medicine, Louisiana State University, Baton Rouge, LA.

PARASITE: *Cryptosporidium* **spp.** (Figure 1.159)

Taxonomy: Protozoan (coccidia). Avian species of this genus include *C. baileyi* and *C. meleagridis*. The latter species has been found to be infective for humans and some other mammals, as well as birds.

Geographic Distribution: Worldwide.

Location in Host: Gastrointestinal, respiratory, and/or urinary tracts depending on host.

Life Cycle: Infection of the bird host follows ingestion of the infective oocyst. Development and reproduction occur in the epithelial cells of the gastrointestinal and respiratory tract primarily. In some bird species, the urinary tract is affected.

Laboratory Diagnosis: Oocysts can be detected with the Sheather's sugar flotation procedure. Acid-fast or other staining procedures of fecal smears can also be used, as well as fecal immunodiagnostic tests.

Size: 4–6 μm in diameter

Clinical Importance: Depending on the body systems affected, birds may show diarrhea, coughing, sneezing, and dyspnea or renal disease. Severe infection may cause death. *Cryptosporidium meleagridis* can infect humans.

PARASITE: **Gastrointestinal Flagellates** (Figures 1.160–1.161, see also 1.32–1.38 for illustrations of *Giardia*)

Taxonomy: Protozoa (flagellates). Several genera are found in the avian digestive tract, including *Trichomonas, Cochlosoma, Histomonas, Giardia, Spironucleus* (= *Hexamita*), and *Chilomastix*.

Geographic Distribution: Worldwide.

Location in Host: *Trichomonas gallinae* is found in the upper digestive system, *Histomonas* in the cecum and liver, and *Cochlosoma, Giardia,* and *Spironucleus* in the intestines.

Life Cycle: Most avian flagellates have only a trophozoite stage. They are transmitted from bird to bird by direct contact and contaminated food or water. Feeding of young birds by adults can also transmit *Trichomonas gallinae,* while *Histomonas* can be carried in the eggs of the cecal roundworm, *Heterakis. Giardia* trophozoites encyst in the intestinal tract. Cysts passed in the feces are ingested by birds. *Chilomastix* also forms cysts.

Laboratory Diagnosis: *Trichomonas* trophozoites have anterior flagella and an undulating membrane. They can usually be detected in smears made from exudates or lesions in the oral cavity, esophagus, and crop. *Giardia* cysts can be recovered by $ZnSO_4$ centrifugal flotation. *Chilomastix* cysts are rarely found in feces. *Giardia, Spironucleus,* and *Cochlosoma* trophozoites may be seen in very fresh fecal smears. *Spironucleus* has no sucking disk, unlike *Giardia* and *Cochlosoma. Histomonas* is unlikely to be detected in fecal smears.

Size:	*Trichomonas*	8–14 μm in length, depending on species
	Giardia trophozoites	10–20 × 5–15 μm
	Giardia cysts	10–14 × 8–10 μm
	Cochlosoma	6–10 × 4–6.5 μm
	Spironucleus	5–12 × 2–7 μm
	Chilomastix	6–24 × 3–10 μm

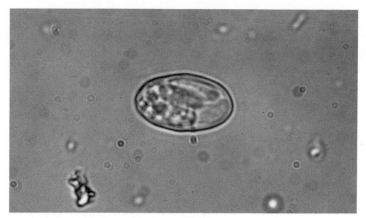

Fig. 1.158. *Sarcocystis* is another coccidian genus that may be found in the feces of carnivorous birds that act as the definitive host of the parasite. Oocysts sporulate in the host, and small sporocysts (approx. 10–12 μm) are passed in the feces.

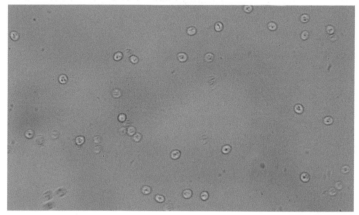

Fig. 1.159. *Cryptosporidium* spp. oocysts in birds are similar in appearance to those of mammalian species. Slides should be examined using the 40× lens of the microscope.

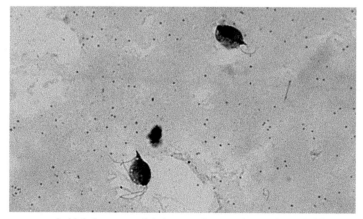

Fig. 1.160. *Trichomonas* spp. in birds have an undulating membrane and several anterior flagella. They can be seen in smears made from lesions in the upper GI tract. The presence of caseous lesions in the esophagus and crop is also helpful in diagnosis.

(Flagellates *continued*)

Clinical Importance: Pigeons and raptors are particularly susceptible to trichomoniasis of the upper digestive tract. Affected birds may show depression and weakness with characteristic plaques and accumulation of cheesy material in the mouth, esophagus, and crop. Severe infections may be fatal. Although many *Giardia* infections are asymptomatic, the parasite can cause diarrhea, depression, and debilitation, particularly in young psittacines. Feather picking associated with infection has also been described. *Histomonas* is the cause of Blackhead in turkeys. Other flagellates may also produce diarrhea, but many infections are asymptomatic. None of these avian flagellates has zoonotic importance.

Helminth Parasites

PARASITE: Avian Ascarids (Figures 1.162–1.163)
Common name: Roundworm, cecal worm (*Heterakis*).

Taxonomy: Nematodes (order Ascaridida). *Ascaridia* spp. and *Heterakis* spp. are common in poultry and many wild bird hosts. *Porrocecum* spp. and *Contracecum* spp. are also found in a variety of bird hosts.

Geographic Distribution: Worldwide.

Location in Host: Intestinal tract; *Heterakis* spp. parasitize the ceca of birds.

Life Cycle: Eggs are passed in the feces of the bird host and develop to the infective stage in the environment. Birds become infected when they ingest infective eggs. Earthworms may act as transport hosts.

Laboratory Diagnosis: Thick-shelled eggs are detected with flotation procedures. Eggs of *Ascaridia* and *Heterakis* are similar in size and morphology and are not easily differentiated.

Size:	*Ascaridia*	77–94 × 43–55 μm
	Heterakis	66–79 × 41–48 μm

Clinical Importance: Larvae of *Ascaridia* appear to be the most pathogenic stage and may cause enteritis in the prepatent period. Heavy burdens of adult worms can cause enteritis and intestinal obstruction. *Heterakis* is primarily important in poultry as a vector of *Histomonas meleagridis* (Blackhead), which can be a serious disease of turkeys. The protozoan is carried from bird to bird in the eggs and larvae of *Heterakis*. Fatal infections of *Heterakis isolonche* due to nodular typhlitis have been reported in pheasants.

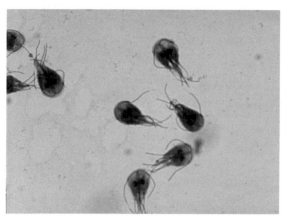

Fig. 1.161. *Giardia* trophozoites found in smears of avian feces are very similar in appearance to these mammalian parasites.

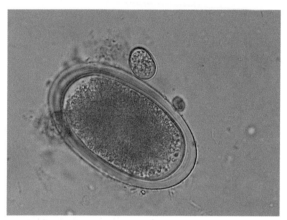

Fig. 1.162. A smooth, thick shell is seen in both *Ascaridia* spp. and *Heterakis* spp. eggs. This sample from a chicken shows both an ascarid egg and a much smaller *Eimeria* oocyst.

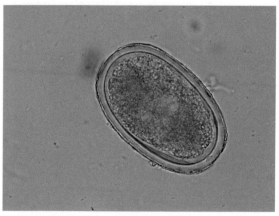

Fig. 1.163. *Ascaridia* egg from a peacock. Another ascarid genus found in ducks and wild birds is *Porrocecum,* which has eggs with a rough shell similar in appearance to that of many mammalian ascarid species.

PARASITE: *Capillaria* **spp.** (Figures 1.164–1.165, 1.167)

Taxonomy: Nematode (order Enoplida). A variety of species can be found in domestic and wild birds.

Geographic Distribution: Worldwide.

Location in Host: Various locations in the gastrointestinal tract, depending on species.

Life Cycle: Eggs are passed in the feces of the host and become infective in the environment. Some species, such as *C. obsignata,* have a direct life cycle, while others have been shown to use an earthworm intermediate host.

Laboratory Diagnosis: Bipolar-plugged eggs can be detected in the feces with flotation techniques.

Size: approx. 45–70 μm in length, depending on species

Clinical Importance: *Capillaria* spp. can cause severe inflammation wherever species occur in the digestive tract, including esophagus, crop, and intestines. Heavy infections may be fatal.

PARASITE: *Trichostrongylus tenuis*, *Amidostomum* **spp., and Other Avian Strongylids** (Figure 1.166)

Taxonomy: Nematodes (order Strongylida). *Trichostrongylus tenuis* and *Amidostomum* occur in domestic and game birds.

Geographic Distribution: Worldwide.

Location in Host: Cecum and intestines of game birds, poultry, and wild birds.

Life Cycle: Eggs are passed from the host in the feces. First-stage larvae hatch from the eggs, develop to the infective stage in the environment, and develop to the adult stage when ingested by the avian host.

Laboratory Diagnosis: Typical thin-shelled strongylid eggs can be detected with flotation procedures.

Size: varies with species
T. tenuis eggs	65–75 μm × 35–42 μm
A. anseri eggs	85–110 × 50–82 μm

Clinical Importance: Heavy infections of *Trichostrongylus tenuis* can produce severe enteritis with resulting hemorrhagic diarrhea, weight loss, and death.

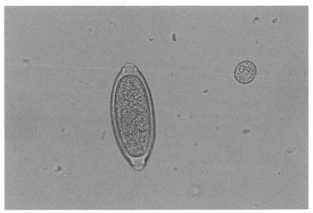

Fig. 1.164. Eggs of *Capillaria* spp. are very common in the feces of domestic and wild birds. The bipolar-plugged eggs have a thick shell and are typically yellowish. This *Capillaria* egg and *Eimeria* oocyst were present in a fecal sample from a backyard chicken flock. *Capillaria* spp. are uncommon in poultry maintained in total-confinement systems.

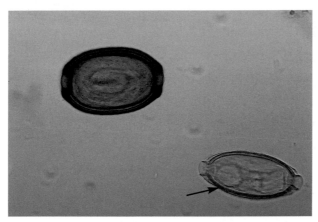

Fig. 1.165. *Capillaria* sp. egg in an owl (*arrow*). The larger, browner egg belongs to *Trichosomoides* sp., a parasite of the bladder of rats. Because parasite eggs of prey are sometimes found in predator feces, it is important to appreciate the normal array of parasites found in a host so spurious parasites can be correctly identified. Photo courtesy of Dr. Stephen Smith, Virginia-Maryland Regional College of Veterinary Medicine, Virginia Tech, Blacksburg, VA.

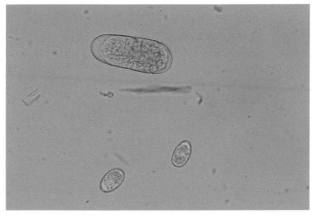

Fig. 1.166. Strongylid egg and coccidia oocysts in an avian fecal sample.

PARASITE: *Syngamus* **spp.** (Figures 1.167–1.168)
                Common name: Gapeworm.

Taxonomy: Nematode (order Strongylida).

Geographic Distribution: Worldwide.

Location in Host: Trachea and bronchi of numerous domestic and wild birds. Species of a similar genus, *Cyathostoma*, are found in some aquatic birds and birds of prey.

Life Cycle: Eggs are produced by females in the trachea and are coughed up, swallowed, and passed out of the host in the feces. Infective larvae may be eaten directly from the environment by the avian host or they may be ingested by an earthworm or molluscan transport host that is eaten, in turn, by a bird.

Laboratory Diagnosis: Ellipsoidal, bipolar eggs are seen in the feces with flotation procedures.

   Size: 80–110 μm × 40–50 μm

Clinical Importance: Young birds are most severely affected. Large numbers of parasites and exudate obstruct the airways and can suffocate the host. The parasite's common name originates from the gaping and gasping of infected birds as they attempt to breathe. *Syngamus* is uncommon in total-confinement poultry systems.

PARASITE: ***Dispharynx, Echinuria, Tetrameres, Subulura, Cheilospirura (Acuaria), Serratospiculum,*** **and Others** (Figures 1.169–1.170)

Taxonomy: Nematodes (order Spirurida).

Geographic Distribution: Worldwide.

Location in Host: Species are found throughout the digestive tract. *Serratospiculum* parasitizes the respiratory tract of some wild birds.

Life Cycle: Adults (except *Serratospiculum*) are located in the digestive tract. Eggs are passed in the feces and are ingested by various arthropod intermediate hosts. Birds are infected by ingesting an intermediate host carrying infective larvae.

Laboratory Diagnosis: Flotation and sedimentation techniques can be used to detect the relatively small, larvated eggs in feces.

   Size: approx. 30–55 × 20–35 μm, depending on species

Clinical Importance: Most infections with this group of parasites are not highly pathogenic. However, *Tetrameres* and *Dispharynx* in large numbers in the proventriculus may cause weight loss and reduced production. In poultry, members of this group of parasites are rare in total-confinement management systems.

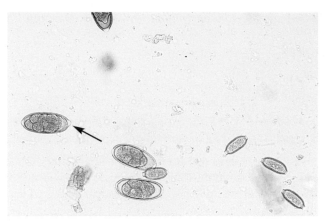

Fig. 1.167. *Syngamus* eggs have bipolar plugs like the eggs of *Capillaria* spp. However, the eggs of *Syngamus* are larger and contain several well-defined cells (morula) when passed in the feces. In this specimen, both *Syngamus* and *Capillaria* eggs are present. The polar plugs of *Syngamus* can be seen in some of the eggs (*arrow*). Photo courtesy of Dr. Robert Ridley, College of Veterinary Medicine, Kansas State University, Manhattan, KS.

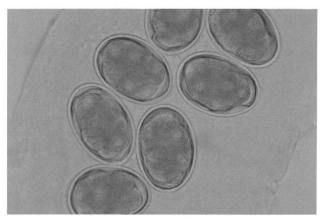

Fig. 1.168. *Cyathostoma bronchialis* is a species similar to *Syngamus* that is found in the respiratory system of some aquatic birds. Other species parasitize raptors. The polar plugs in this species are not prominent. The eggs shown here are inside the uterus of a female worm removed from a goose.

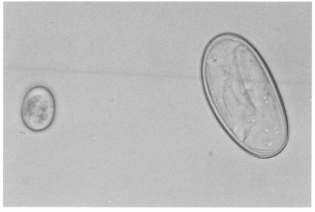

Fig. 1.169. *Tetrameres* egg in the feces of a homing pigeon. Like other spirurid eggs, this *Tetrameres* egg is larvated when passed in the feces, but further specific identification is difficult. Also pictured is a coccidia oocyst. Photo courtesy of Dr. Robert Ridley, College of Veterinary Medicine, Kansas State University, Manhattan, KS.

PARASITE: *Echinostoma* **spp.**, *Echinoparyphium*, *Prosthogonimus* **spp., and Others** (Figures 1.171–1.172)

        Common name: Fluke.

Taxonomy: Trematode.

Geographic Distribution: Worldwide.

Location in Host: Domestic and wild birds are parasitized by many fluke species. Adults can be found in various body systems, including the intestines and respiratory and reproductive tracts.

Life Cycle: Adult worms produce eggs that leave the host principally via the digestive tract. The first intermediate host is a mollusk, and a variety of animals act as second intermediate host depending on the fluke species (with the exception of schistosome flukes, which do not require a second intermediate host).

Laboratory Diagnosis: Fluke eggs in feces are best detected with a sedimentation technique because of their higher density. Fluke eggs are typically operculated and brown.

    Size: highly variable with species, approx. 20–100 µm in length

Clinical Importance: Many fluke infections are of low pathogenicity. Some genera of importance in domestic poultry are *Echinostoma* and *Echinoparyphium,* which may cause enteritis, and *Prosthogonimus,* a parasite of the oviduct, which can cause abnormal egg production and peritonitis. Because of their complex life cycles, flukes will be seen only in birds with access to intermediate hosts and will not occur in confinement poultry operations.

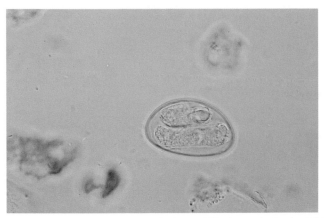

Fig. 1.170. Spirurid egg in the feces of a red-tailed hawk. The larva within the egg is clearly visible. Photo courtesy of Dr. Stephen Smith, Virginia-Maryland Regional College of Veterinary Medicine, Virginia Tech, Blacksburg, VA.

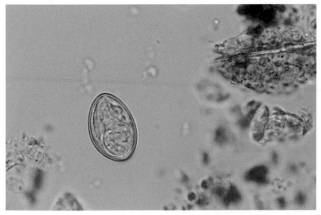

Fig. 1.171. Fluke egg in the feces of a screech owl. The operculum is easily seen (*arrow*).

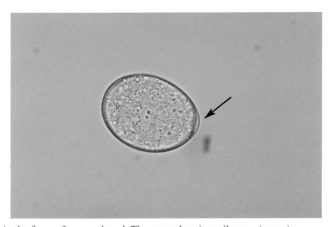

Fig. 1.172. The developing miracidium can be seen inside this avian trematode egg found in feces from a bird of prey.

PARASITE: *Davainea* **spp.,** *Choanotaenia* **spp.,** *Raillietina* **spp.,** *Hymenolepis* **spp., and Others** (Figures 1.173–1.175)

> Common name: Tapeworm.

Taxonomy: Cestodes.

Geographic Distribution: Worldwide.

Location in Host: Small intestine of a wide variety of domestic and wild birds.

Life Cycle: Eggs are passed in the feces. Insects are the most common intermediate hosts, but other invertebrates may also be used by some species (e.g., the intermediate host of *Davainea* is a mollusk).

Laboratory Diagnosis: Although proglottids are intermittently passed in the feces, detection of eggs by fecal exam is unreliable, and diagnosis is usually made at necropsy.

> Size: varies with species; individual eggs of many species are approx. 50–80 μm; some species have large egg packets

Clinical Importance: Many tapeworm infections are asymptomatic. However, some are serious pathogens; for example, *Davainea proglottina* and *Raillietina echinobothrida* can cause severe enteritis and death in domestic poultry. Tapeworms are common in unconfined poultry with access to the intermediate hosts.

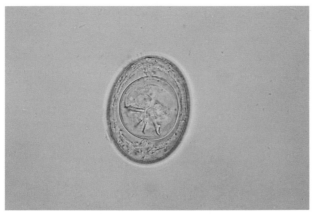

Fig. 1.173. Avian tapeworm egg. Several embryonic hooks are clearly visible, and this characteristic is very helpful in identification. Photo courtesy of Dr. Stephen Smith, Virginia-Maryland Regional College of Veterinary Medicine, Virginia Tech, Blacksburg, VA.

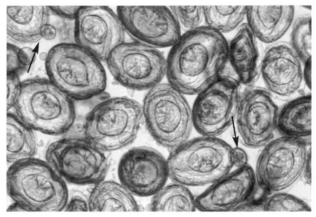

Fig. 1.174. Tapeworm eggs from a magpie. Scattered among the cestode eggs are occasional coccidia oocysts (*arrows*). Photo courtesy of Dr. Alvin Gajadhar, Centre for Animal Parasitology, CFIA, Saskatoon, Saskatchewan, Canada.

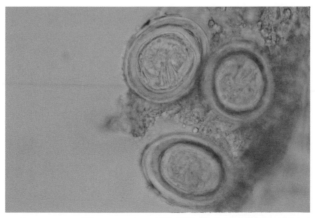

Fig. 1.175. Tapeworm eggs from a canary. Photo courtesy of Dr. Ellis Greiner, College of Veterinary Medicine, University of Florida, Gainesville, FL.

PARASITE: *Polymorphus* **spp.,** *Filicollis* **spp., and Others** (Figures 1.176–1.177)
Common name: Thorny-headed worm.

Taxonomy: Acanthocephalan.

Geographic Distribution: Worldwide.

Location in Host: Digestive system.

Life Cycle: Eggs are passed in the feces of the host. Infective larvae develop in arthropod intermediate hosts and infect birds when they are ingested.

Laboratory Diagnosis: Eggs are not consistently recovered by flotation procedures. A sedimentation procedure should also be performed.

Size: approx. 50–100 μm in length, depending on species

Clinical Importance: Thorny-headed worms are primarily parasites of free-ranging and wild birds because of their complex life cycles. Heavy infections may cause diarrhea and debilitation.

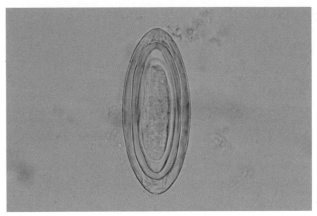

Fig. 1.176. Egg of a thorny-headed worm (*Centrorhynchus*) from the feces of a barred owl. Acanthocephalan eggs have several internal layers surrounding the larva (acanthor). Photo courtesy of Dr. Ellis Greiner, College of Veterinary Medicine, University of Florida, Gainesville, FL.

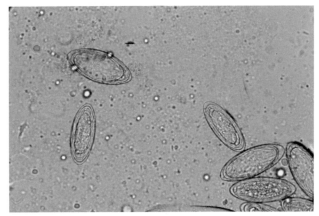

Fig. 1.177. Acanthocephalan eggs in the feces of a blue jay. Photo courtesy of Dr. Thomas Nolan, School of Veterinary Medicine, University of Pennsylvania, Philadelphia, PA.

Rodents and Rabbits

Protozoan Parasites

PARASITE: *Eimeria* spp. (Figures 1.178–1.180)
       Common name: Coccidia.

Taxonomy: Protozoan (coccidia).

Geographic Distribution: Worldwide.

Location in Host: A variety of species parasitize the intestinal tract of rodents and rabbits. *Eimeria stiedae* is found in the bile ducts of rabbits.

Life Cycle: Oocysts passed in the feces can sporulate quickly and infect the host when ingested. Asexual and sexual reproduction occurs in cells of the gastrointestinal tract.

Laboratory Diagnosis: Oocysts can be detected in feces by centrifugal or simple flotation techniques. Oocysts are elliptical to spherical shaped.

     Size: approx. 10–45 × 10–30 μm, depending on species

Clinical Importance: Some species are nonpathogenic. Pathogenic intestinal coccidia can cause anorexia, weight loss, profuse diarrhea, and death. *Eimeria stiedae* infection of the rabbit liver can cause anorexia, diarrhea, distended abdomen, and death.

     Rodents may also be infected with species of *Giardia* and *Cryptosporidium* (see Figs. 1.32–1.38, 1.29).

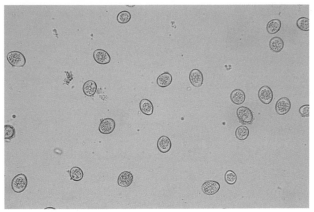

Fig. 1.178. *Eimeria* oocysts have smooth, clear cyst walls and contain a single round cell when freshly passed. The oocysts in this Fig. are *Eimeria nieschulzi*, a parasite of rats. Photo courtesy of Dr. George Conder, Pfizer Veterinary Medicine Pharmaceuticals Clinical Development, Pfizer, Inc., Kalamazoo, MI.

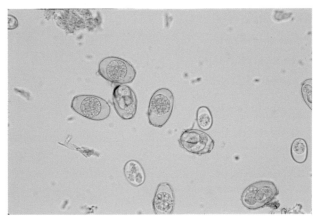

Fig. 1.179. Rodent and rabbit hosts may be infected with multiple species of coccidia. Oocysts of more than one species of rabbit *Eimeria* were detected in this sample.

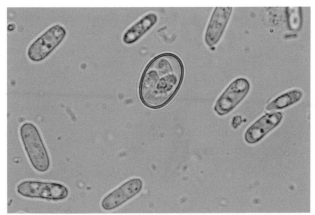

Fig. 1.180. Once in the environment, oocysts undergo sporulation to the infective stage. Sporulated oocysts of *Eimeria* contain four sporocysts, each containing two sporozoites (individual organisms). The sporocysts can clearly be seen inside this rabbit *Eimeria* sp. oocyst. Surrounding the oocyst are several elongated nonpathogenic yeast organisms that are very common in rabbit feces.

Helminth Parasites

PARASITE: *Syphacia obvelata* (Figure 1.181)
        Common name: Pinworm.

Taxonomy: Nematode (order Oxyurida).

Geographic Distribution: Worldwide.

Location in Host: Large intestine of mice and gerbils.

Life Cycle: Eggs passed in the feces quickly become infective. Rodents develop infection following ingestion of larvated eggs.

Laboratory Diagnosis: When present in the feces, eggs can be detected by routine flotation techniques. Eggs are normally found on the skin in the perineal region of infected animals.

    Size: 100–142 × 30–40 μm

Clinical Importance: Infections are typically subclinical.

PARASITE: *Aspicularis tetraptera* (Figure 1.182)
        Common name: Pinworm.

Taxonomy: Nematode (order Oxyurida).

Geographic Distribution: Worldwide.

Location in Host: Large intestine of mice.

Life Cycle: The life cycle is similar to that of *Syphacia oblevata*. Adult pinworms develop following ingestion of infective eggs.

Laboratory Diagnosis: Eggs can be detected in feces by centrifugal or simple flotation techniques. The eggs are ellipsoidal with a distinctive double shell wall and contain an undifferentiated embryo in fresh feces.

    Size: 70–98 × 29–50 μm

Clinical Importance: Infections are usually subclinical.

PARASITE: *Passalurus ambiguus* (Figure 1.183)
        Common name: Pinworm.

Taxonomy: Nematode (order Oxyurida).

Geographic Distribution: Worldwide.

Location in Host: Cecum of rabbits.

Life Cycle: Eggs are passed in the feces of infected rabbits. The eggs become infective within a short period and infect the next host when ingested.

Laboratory Diagnosis: Eggs can be detected in feces by flotation techniques. The eggs have a smooth, clear shell wall that is flat on one side.

    Size: 95–103 × 43 μm

Clinical Importance: Infections are usually subclinical.

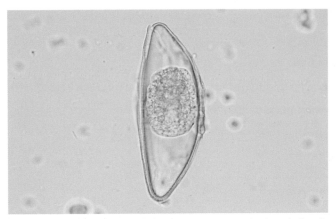

Fig. 1.181. *Syphacia* egg in feces from a gerbil. Eggs of *Syphacia* have a smooth, clear shell wall, are flat on one side, and contain an undifferentiated morula in fresh fecal samples.

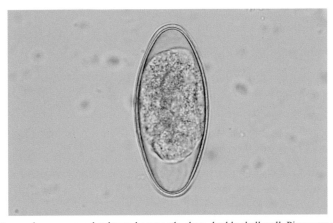

Fig. 1.182. *Aspicularis* eggs have narrowed poles and a smooth, clear, double shell wall. Pinworms are common in rodents.

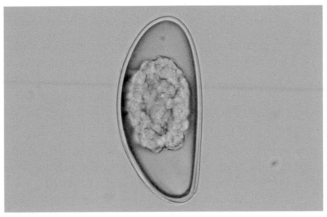

Fig. 1.183. *Passalurus ambiguus* eggs have an operculum-like structure at one end, and the eggs contain an undifferentiated morula in fresh fecal samples.

PARASITE: *Paraspidodera uncinata, Heterakis spumosa* (Figure 1.184)

Taxonomy: Nematodes (order Ascaridida).

Geographic Distribution: Worldwide.

Location in Host: Cecum of guinea pigs (*Paraspidodera*) and rats (*Heterakis*).

Life Cycle: Eggs passed in the feces develop to the infective stage and infect the host when they are ingested.

Laboratory Diagnosis: Fecal flotation procedures can be used to recover these thick-shelled eggs.

Size:	*Heterakis*	55–60 × 40–55 μm
	Paraspidodera	43 × 31 μm

Clinical Importance: Infection is usually subclinical. These parasites are seen primarily in wild rats and guinea pigs raised on dirt.

PARASITE: *Heligosomoides polygyrus, Nippostrongylus braziliensis, Obeliscoides cuniculi, Graphidium strigosum* (Figure 1.185)

Taxonomy: Nematodes (order Strongylida).

Geographic Distribution: Worldwide.

Location in Host: Stomach (*Obeliscoides, Graphidium*) of rabbits; small intestine of rats (*Nippostrongylus*) and mice (*Heligosomoides*).

Life Cycle: Eggs passed in the feces develop into first-stage larvae, which hatch and continue development in the environment. In most cases, the definitive host is infected by ingesting third-stage larvae, but larvae of *Nippostrongylus braziliensis* usually penetrate the skin of the final host.

Laboratory Diagnosis: Fecal flotation procedures will recover the typical strongylid eggs produced by these parasites.

Size: 52–106 × 28–58 μm (eggs), depending on species

Clinical Importance: Parasites belonging to this group of nematodes are unlikely to occur in caged rabbits and rodents but are common in wild animals. Infection is usually subclinical.

PARASITE: *Hymenolepis* **spp.** (Figures 1.186–1.187)
        Common name: Dwarf tapeworm of humans (*Hymenolepis nana*).

Taxonomy: Cestode. The most common species in domestic rodents is *Hymenolepis* (= *Vampirolepis*) *nana*. Other species infecting rodents are *H. diminuta* and *H. microstoma*.

Geographic Distribution: Worldwide.

Location in Host: Small intestine of rodents (mouse, rat, hamster). Humans and other primates also serve as hosts for *H. nana*.

Life Cycle: Eggs passed in the feces of definitive hosts are ingested by beetle intermediate hosts. Rodents and humans are infected following ingestion of the intermediate host containing cysticercoids. Infection with adult *H. nana* can also follow ingestion of the egg.

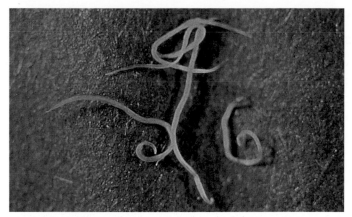

Fig. 1.184. Specimens of *Paraspidodera uncinata*, the cecal worm of guinea pigs. The eggs produced by this cecal nematode of rodents are similar to those of the avian cecal worm, *Heterakis* (Fig. 1.162). Photo courtesy of Dr. David Baker, School of Veterinary Medicine, Louisiana State University, Baton Rouge, LA.

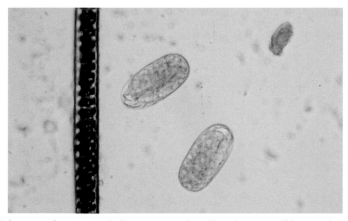

Fig. 1.185. These *Heligosomoides* eggs are similar to eggs produced by other strongylid nematodes of rabbits and rodents. Photo courtesy of Dr. David Baker, School of Veterinary Medicine, Louisiana State University, Baton Rouge, LA.

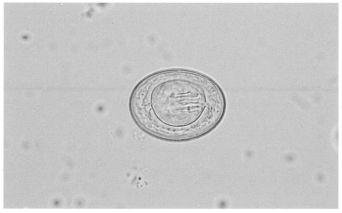

Fig. 1.186. *Hymenolepis nana* infects rodents and primates. Eggs are elliptical in shape with a smooth, clear shell wall and contain an embryo with six hooks. There are two knoblike protrusions at each end of the embryo. Like eggs of other common tapeworms, hooks are visible within the embryo.

139

Hymenolepis (*continued*)

Laboratory Diagnosis: Eggs with 6 embryonic hooks are detected by either centrifugal or simple fecal flotation examination.

Size:	*H. nana*	40–45 × 34–37 μm
	H. diminuta	60–88 × 52–81 μm

Clinical Importance: Infections are usually subclinical. Heavy infections, particularly in young animals, can result in poor growth and rarely intestinal impaction and death.

PARASITE: *Cittotaenia* **spp.** (Figure 1.188)
Common name: Rabbit tapeworm.

Taxonomy: Cestode.

Geographic Distribution: Worldwide.

Location in Host: Small intestine of rabbits and hares.

Life Cycle: Eggs are ingested by free-living oribatid mites and develop into the cysticercoid larval stage. Rabbits are infected when they ingest the infected mites.

Laboratory Diagnosis: Fecal flotation procedures will recover *Cittotaenia* eggs.

Size: 64 μm in diameter

Clinical Importance: Heavy infections may cause weight loss.

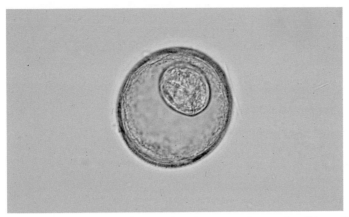

Fig. 1.187. Other species of *Hymenolepis* found in rodents have larger, rounder eggs than *H. nana*. Hymenolepid eggs are seen occasionally in fecal samples of dogs and cats that have recently eaten rodents.

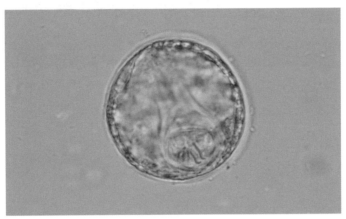

Fig. 1.188. *Cittotaenia* eggs are quite similar in appearance to *Hymenolepis* eggs. The hooks in the tapeworm embryo are usually easily seen.

Reptiles

PARASITE: *Entamoeba, Cryptosporidium, Eimeria, Isospora,* and *Caryospora* (Figures 1.189–1.191, 1.93)

Taxonomy: Protozoa.

Geographic Distribution: Worldwide.

Location in Host: Gastrointestinal tract.

Life Cycle: Reptiles are infected by ingestion of cysts (*Entamoeba*) or oocysts that are passed in host feces.

Laboratory Diagnosis: *Eimeria, Caryospora,* and *Cryptosporidium* oocysts can be detected by fecal flotation techniques (the centrifugal flotation procedure with Sheather's sugar solution is recommended for *Cryptosporidium*). Wet mounts of feces or colonic washings can be examined for *Entamoeba* trophozoites and cysts. Fecal smears may also be stained with Wright's stain or Giemsa stain.

Clinical Importance: *Cryptosporidium serpentis* may cause chronic hypertrophic gastritis in snakes, associated with weight loss and regurgitation. *Entamoeba invadens* can cause bloody diarrhea and hepatitis in snakes and some tortoise and lizard hosts. Weight loss and enteritis may accompany infection with *Eimeria* (all reptiles) and *Caryospora* (primarily snakes).

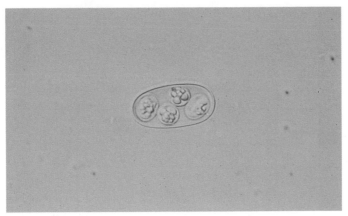

Fig. 1.189. Sporulated *Eimeria* oocyst in the feces of a king snake. Oocysts of prey coccidia species may also be found in the feces of carnivorous reptiles. Photo courtesy of Dr. Robert Ridley, College of Veterinary Medicine, Kansas State University, Manhattan, KS.

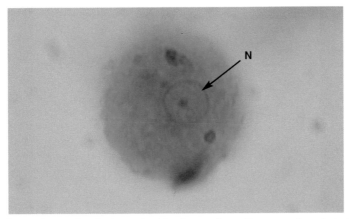

Fig. 1.190. *Entamoeba invadens* trophozoite in a stained fecal smear from a Burmese python. A single nucleus (N) is seen in the trophozoite. Trophozoite movement can be seen in a wet mount of fresh feces. Photo courtesy of Dr. Ellis Greiner, College of Veterinary Medicine, University of Florida, Gainesville, FL.

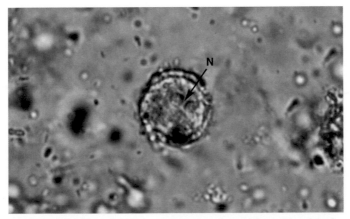

Fig. 1.191. Cyst of *Entamoeba invadens* in an iodine-stained smear of reptile feces. Two of the four nuclei (N) present in the cyst can be seen (*arrow*). Photo courtesy of Dr. Thomas Nolan, School of Veterinary Medicine, University of Pennsylvania, Philadelphia, PA.

143

PARASITE: Reptile Helminths (Figures 1.192–1.199)

Taxonomy: Nematodes, cestodes (tapeworms), trematodes (flukes), acanthocephalans (thorny-headed worms), and pentastomid parasites.

Geographic Distribution: Worldwide.

Location in Host: Helminth parasites can be found in a variety of body systems, although those detected by fecal exam are primarily gastrointestinal or respiratory system parasites.

Life Cycle: Life cycle varies widely depending on the species. Some nematodes have a direct life cycle. Other nematodes and the remaining helminth groups all require at least one intermediate host.

Laboratory Diagnosis: Eggs are detected in feces by flotation or sedimentation procedures.

Clinical Importance: As in other hosts, low levels of helminth infection are usually well tolerated by reptiles. Heavy infections may result in clinical disease, especially in young or immunosuppressed animals. The complex life cycles of most flukes, tapeworms, and thorny-headed worms make these parasites uncommon in reptiles bred in captivity.

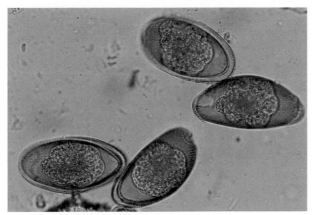

Fig. 1.192. Pinworm eggs are frequently encountered in reptile feces. These eggs are usually elongated and may appear flat on one side. The eggs shown here are from a bearded dragon.

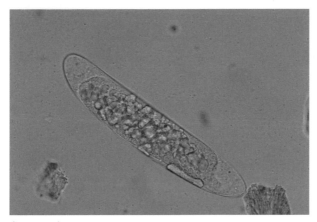

Fig. 1.193. Pinworm egg from a turtle.

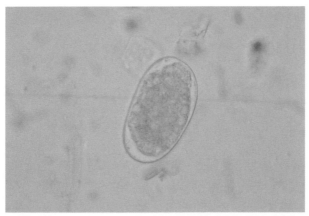

Fig. 1.194. *Kalicephalus* sp. egg from a python. This is one of the genera of strongylid nematodes parasitizing reptiles. Eggs of this nematode group are thin shelled. In fresh feces reptile strongylid eggs may be larvated or contain a morula (cluster of cells), like the one shown here. Photo courtesy of Dr. Ellis Greiner, College of Veterinary Medicine, University of Florida, Gainesville, FL.

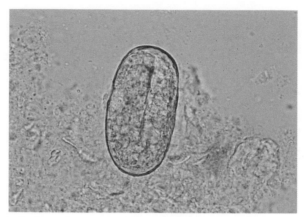

Fig. 1.195. *Rhabdias* egg in the feces of a rat snake. Eggs containing a larva are passed in the feces and are smaller than strongylid eggs.

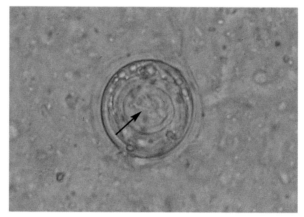

Fig. 1.196. Tapeworm egg from a water moccasin snake. This egg is surrounded by a gelatinous layer with one hook of the hexacanth embryo visible (*arrow*).

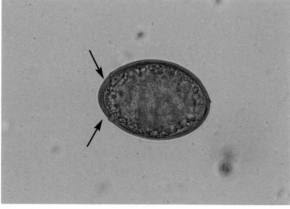

Fig. 1.197. Fluke (trematode) infections are common in wild reptiles, especially those associated with water. The operculum is clearly visible (*arrows*) in this fluke egg from a turtle.

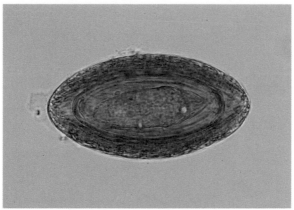

Fig. 1.198. Acanthocephalan (thorny-headed worms) are also common in wild reptiles. This egg was found in mammalian feces but shows the complex layered shell that would also be seen in the eggs of thorny-headed worms of snakes.

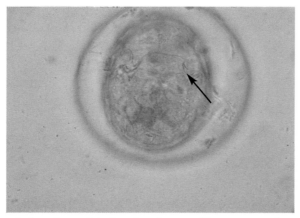

Fig. 1.199. Pentastomid egg in feces from a Bolen's python. Pentastomids are an unusual group that shows some arthropod characteristics. Adults are parasites of the respiratory tract. Large eggs (over 100 μm) passed in the feces are often surrounded by a capsule. Larvae within the eggs have legs bearing hooklets (*arrow*) and could be mistaken for mite eggs. An intermediate host is required for completion of the life cycle. Photo courtesy of Dr. Ellis Greiner, College of Veterinary Medicine, University of Florida, Gainesville, FL.

Detection of Protozoan and Helminth Parasites in the Urinary, Reproductive, and Integumentary Systems and in the Eye

TECHNIQUES FOR PARASITE RECOVERY

Parasites of the Urinary System

Several organisms parasitize the urinary tract, and their eggs and cysts can be detected by routine urine sedimentation. Samples collected by cystocentesis are preferred because voided urine samples could be contaminated with fecal material containing parasite eggs or larvae from the intestinal or respiratory systems.

Urine Sedimentation

1. Centrifuge 5–10 ml of urine in a conical-tip centrifuge tube for 5 minutes at 1500–2000 rpm (approximately 100 G).
2. Decant the supernatant fluid, leaving 0.5 ml. Resuspend the sediment.
3. Transfer a drop of sediment to a slide, add a coverslip, and examine.

Parasites of the Reproductive Tract

Parasites of the reproductive tract are not important pathogens of common domestic species in North America, with the exception of *Tritrichomonas foetus*. This parasite of cattle is found in the uterus and vagina of cows and the prepuce of bulls. Diagnosis of infection is usually by identification of the organisms in preputial samples from bulls, although vaginal or cervical secretions from cows can also be tested. It is recommended that samples be collected in lactated Ringer's solution and submitted to a laboratory for culture in Diamond's medium. There is also a commercial kit available that provides a plastic pouch containing medium into which the sample can be inoculated and cultured (InPouch® TF, BioMed Diagnostics, Inc., Santa Clara, CA 95054, www.biomed1.com).

Bovine Preputial Sample Collection

1. Attach a dry 21-inch infusion pipette to a 20 cc syringe and insert into the prepuce of the bull. The tip of the pipette is scraped back and forth across the epithelium while suction is applied.
2. Examine the collected sample microscopically immediately if desired and then inoculate into Ringer's solution (or the commercial InPouch®) and refrigerate for transport to the laboratory for culture.
3. Samples not placed directly into nutritive medium should not be held for more than 48 hours in Ringer's or other balanced-salt solution.

Helminth Parasites of the Integumentary System

Several filarid nematode parasites produce microfilariae that are found in the subcutaneous tissue. These larvae can be detected in fresh skin biopsies or on examination of fixed and stained biopsy tissue sections. For recovery of microfilariae from fresh biopsies, the biopsy is macerated and allowed to incubate in saline for several hours at room temperature. Following incubation, the saline is examined microscopically for the presence of microfilariae. Free-living nematodes that occasionally invade skin may also be seen in fresh or fixed and stained skin biopsies.

URINARY SYSTEM PARASITES

PARASITE: *Pearsonema (= Capillaria) plica, P. feliscati* (Figures 2.1–2.2)

Taxonomy: Nematode (order Enoplida). These parasites were previously included in the genus *Capillaria.*

Geographic Distribution: Worldwide.

Location in Host: Adult worms in the bladder of dogs and foxes (*P. plica*) and cats (*P. feliscati*).

Life Cycle: Parasite eggs passed in the urine become infective in the environment. Although the life cycle is not known with certainty, the final host is probably infected by ingesting an earthworm intermediate host or a transport host, such as a bird.

Laboratory Diagnosis: Typical capillarid eggs are detected in urine sediment. Cystocentesis is preferred for collecting urine samples since fecal material containing similar eggs of other capillarid species may contaminate voided urine samples.

    Size: 51–65 × 24–32 μm

Clinical Importance: Many infections are asymptomatic, although infected animals may develop cystitis.

PARASITE: *Dioctophyme renale* (Figure 2.3)
        Common name: Giant kidney worm.

Taxonomy: Nematode (order Enoplida).

Geographic Distribution: North America and Europe.

Location in Host: Kidney and occasionally peritoneal cavity of dogs, mink, and other domestic and wild animals.

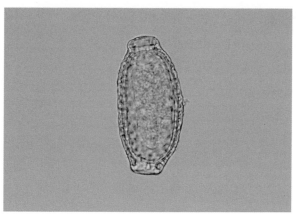

Fig. 2.1. *Pearsonema feliscati* egg in a urine sedimentation procedure. Methylene blue stain is often added to these preparations, which will stain the eggs purple. Like other capillarids, *P. feliscati* eggs are elongated and bipolar plugged.

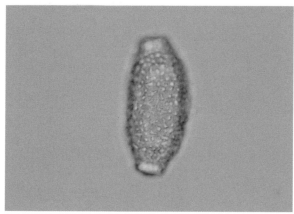

Fig. 2.2. If the microscope is focused on the shell wall of the *Pearsonema* egg, a thick globular pattern of ridges can be seen.

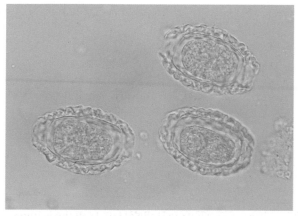

Fig. 2.3. *Dioctophyme* eggs are larger than those of *Pearsonema* and have a thicker eggshell with a rougher surface.

Life Cycle: Adult worms in the kidney produce eggs that are passed in the urine. The first intermediate host is an annelid worm; the second intermediate host is a fish. The final host becomes infected when it eats a fish containing infective parasite larvae.

Laboratory Diagnosis: Eggs with a thick, rough shell are detected in the urine.

Size: 60–80 × 39–46 μm

Clinical Importance: The spectacular adult worms (females may reach 100 cm in length) enter the renal pelvis and eventually destroy the kidney, leaving only the capsule. Typically only one kidney (usually the right) is affected. Most infections are asymptomatic, despite the loss of a kidney, although hematuria and dysuria may occur. *Dioctophyme renale* is a rare finding in dogs in North America.

PARASITE: *Stephanurus dentatus* (Figure 2.4)
          Common name: Kidney worm.

Taxonomy: Nematode (order Strongylida).

Geographic Distribution: Tropical and subtropical regions.

Location in Host: Adults are found in the wall of the ureters and the pelvis of the kidney as well as in the peritoneal fat of swine.

Life Cycle: Parasite eggs leave the host via the urine. Like other strongylids, first-stage larvae of *S. dentatus* hatch from the eggs and develop to the infective third stage. The pig definitive host is infected by ingestion of infective larvae or of an earthworm transport host or by skin penetration by infective larvae. Once in the host, larvae migrate through the liver before moving to the perirenal tissues, where development is completed.

Laboratory Diagnosis: Diagnosis is made by detection of eggs in urine sedimentation tests or from clinical signs. However, disease may be present before the infection is patent (prepatent period is 4–6 months).

Size: 100 × 60 μm

Clinical Importance: The damage associated with larval migration through the liver is an important component of disease caused by the parasite. Pigs may show reduced growth or weight loss and general loss of condition. *Stephanurus dentatus* is unlikely to occur in modern swine confinement systems.

PARASITE: *Trichosomoides crassicauda* (Figures 2.5, 1.165)

Taxonomy: Nematode (order Enoplida).

Geographic Distribution: Worldwide.

Location in Host: Adult female worms are found in the wall of the bladder of wild and laboratory rats. Male worms exist as hyperparasites in the reproductive tract of the females.

Life Cycle: Eggs leave the host in the urine. Infection occurs when eggs are ingested by the host.

Laboratory Diagnosis: Infection is often detected by identification of adults in the bladder or during histologic examination of bladder sections, but diagnosis may also be made by finding eggs in the urine. *Trichosomoides* eggs are brown with bipolar plugs.

Size: 60–70 × 30–35 μm

Clinical Importance: Infection is typically subclinical but is undesirable in laboratory rats.

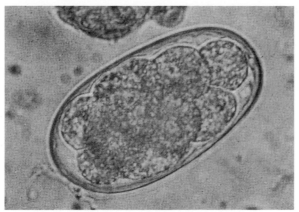

Fig. 2.4. *Stephanurus dentatus* adults produce typical strongylid eggs that can be seen in urine. However, disease may develop before the infection becomes patent. Photo courtesy of Dr. T. Bonner Stewart, School of Veterinary Medicine, Louisiana State University, Baton Rouge, LA.

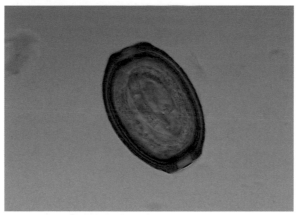

Fig. 2.5. The brown eggs of *Trichosomoides* have bipolar plugs. Photo courtesy of Dr. Stephen Smith, Virginia-Maryland Regional College of Veterinary Medicine, Virginia Tech, Blacksburg, VA.

REPRODUCTIVE SYSTEM PARASITES

PARASITE: *Tritrichomonas foetus* (Figure 2.6)

Taxonomy: Protozoan (flagellate).

Geographic Distribution: Worldwide, but uncommon where artificial insemination is widely practiced.

Location in Host: Preputial cavity of bulls, uterus and vagina of cows.

Life Cycle: Organisms are transmitted during breeding. The trophozoite in the reproductive tract is the only form of the organism.

Laboratory Diagnosis: Organisms are detected in vaginal or uterine discharges or in preputial scrapings. The prepuce is the site most frequently sampled. Organisms may be present in small numbers, and culture is recommended using Diamond's medium or the commercial InPouch® system available in North America. *Tritrichomonas* is easily recognized by its undulating membrane and three anterior flagella. A polymerase chain reaction (PCR) test is also available.

   Size: 10–25 × 3–15 µm

Clinical Importance: The presence of *Tritrichomonas foetus* in a cattle herd produces chronic abortion and infertility and can have a serious economic impact on production.

PARASITES OF OTHER SYSTEMS (EXCLUDING ARTHROPODS)

PARASITE: *Onchocerca* **spp.,** *Stephanofilaria* **spp.** (Figures 2.7–2.8)

Taxonomy: Nematodes (order Spirurida).

Geographic Distribution: *Onchocerca cervicalis* and *O. gutterosa* are found worldwide. Other species have more limited distribution, primarily in Africa but also in the Middle East and Asia. *Stephanofilaria* spp. are found worldwide.

Location in Host: *Onchocerca cervicalis* is found in the equine nuchal ligament. Other species are bovine parasites. *Onchocerca gutterosa* parasitizes the nuchal and gastrosplenic ligament; *O. gibsoni* is found in subcutaneous and intermuscular nodules; and *O. armillata* is found in the wall of the thoracic aorta. *Stephanofilaria* spp. live in the subcutaneous tissue of the ventrum in cattle.

Life Cycle: Depending on the parasite species, *Culicoides* (midges)*, Simulium* (blackflies)*, Haematobia* (horn flies), and *Musca* species act as the intermediate host and transmit the parasite during feeding.

Laboratory Diagnosis: Diagnosis is made by skin biopsy of affected areas and examination for microfilariae following saline incubation or histopathologic examination. Examination of tissues from lesions caused by *Stephanofilaria* will reveal both adults and microfilariae.

   Size: *Onchocerca* microfilariae   approx. 200 to >300 µm in length, depending on species

              Stephanofilaria microfilariae   approx. 50 µm

Clinical Importance: *Onchocerca* spp. are not generally considered to be highly pathogenic parasites, although equine *O. cervicalis* infection can be associated with dermatitis in horses, and some of the bovine species cause skin or connective tissue lesions that must be trimmed at slaughter. In North America, localized ventral midline dermatitis caused by *Stephanofilaria* is relatively common in adult cattle but has no clinical significance.

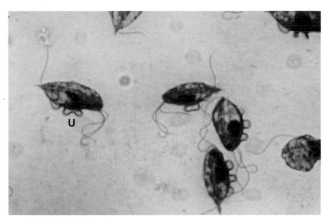

Fig. 2.6. *Tritrichomonas foetus* organisms from culture. The undulating membrane (U) and anterior flagella can be seen in several of the organisms. In culture, living organisms move in a jerky motion and the rippling undulating membrane can be seen with the 40× objective. Photo courtesy of Dr. Alvin Gajadhar, Centre for Animal Parasitology, CFIA, Saskatoon, Saskatchewan, Canada.

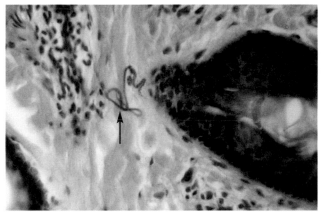

Fig. 2.7. Microfilariae of *Onchocerca gutterosa* (*arrow*) in bovine skin. Diagnosis can be made more rapidly by incubating skin biopsies in saline and examining the fluid several hours later for moving microfilariae that have migrated out of the skin. Photo courtesy of Dr. Fernando Paiva, Universidade Federal de Mato Grosso do Sul, Campo Grande, MS, Brazil.

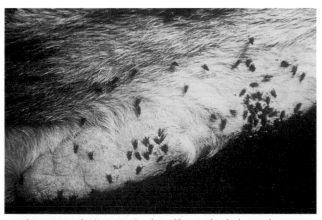

Fig. 2.8. Horn flies (*Haematobia irritans*) feeding on a *Stephanofilaria stilesi* lesion on the ventrum of a bovine host. The flies are the intermediate host of the parasite and ingest microfilariae in the lesion during feeding. *Stephanofilaria stilesi* is common, but unimportant, in North America. Photo courtesy of Dr. Jeffrey F. Williams, Vanson HaloSource, Inc., Redmond, WA.

PARASITE: *Dracunculus insignis* (Figure 2.9)

Taxonomy: Nematode (order Spirurida).

Geographic Distribution: North America.

Location in Host: Adults occur in the subcutaneous tissue, usually on the limbs. Raccoons, other wild animals, and occasionally dogs are infected.

Life Cycle: The female worm creates an ulcer on the skin of a limb. When the limb is placed in water, the female extrudes a portion of the uterus, which ruptures, releasing first-stage larvae into the water. Larvae are ingested by a copepod, *Cyclops,* that acts as the first intermediate host. The definitive host becomes infected by drinking water containing the infected intermediate host.

Laboratory Diagnosis: The diagnosis is usually made by examination of the skin lesion and removal of the worm.

Clinical Importance: *Dracunculus* occurs infrequently in dogs but can cause a chronic ulcer that may develop secondary bacterial infection.

PARASITE: *Pelodera strongyloides* (Figure 2.10)

Taxonomy: Nematode (order Rhabditida).

Geographic Distribution: Worldwide.

Location in Host: Skin.

Life Cycle: *Pelodera strongyloides* is a free-living nematode that may invade the skin of animals. It is usually seen as a pathogen where animals are confined to areas with moist bedding high in organic material that will support growth and development of the nematodes.

Laboratory Diagnosis: Parasite infection can be diagnosed by finding first-stage (rhabditiform) larvae in skin scrapings from affected areas.

Clinical Importance: *Pelodera* is an uncommon cause of dermatitis in a variety of animal species.

PARASITE: *Thelazia* **spp.** (Figure 2.11)
          Common name: Eye worm.

Taxonomy: Nematode (order Spirurida).

Geographic Distribution: Worldwide.

Location in Host: Conjunctival sac and lacrimal duct of cattle, horses, dogs.

Life Cycle: Muscid flies act as intermediate hosts and ingest first-stage larvae released by adult worms into the tears. Development to the third larval stage occurs in the fly, which deposits the infective larvae on the host during feeding.

Laboratory Diagnosis: Laboratory diagnosis is unnecessary since the worms can be seen during examination of the eyes of the host.

    Size: adult worms 1–2 cm

Clinical Importance: Worms may cause tearing and conjunctivitis, but many chronic cases are asymptomatic.

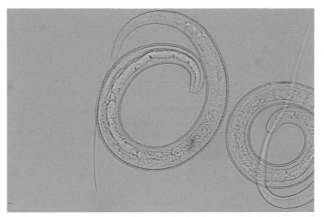

Fig. 2.9. First-stage larvae of *Dracunculus insignis*. These distinctive larvae with their long, thin tails can be teased from the uterus of a worm removed from a skin ulcer and confirm the diagnosis of *Dracunculus* infection.

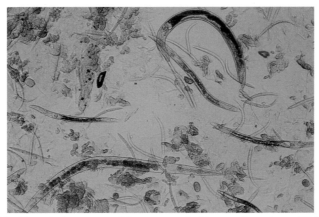

Fig. 2.10. All stages of the life cycle from egg to adult are present in this agar plate culture of *Pelodera*. Only larvae would be present in scrapings of skin infected with this free-living nematode.

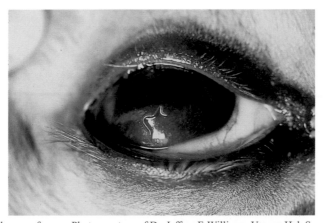

Fig. 2.11. *Thelazia* in the eye of a cow. Photo courtesy of Dr. Jeffrey F. Williams, Vanson HaloSource, Inc., Redmond, WA.

PARASITE: *Besnoitia* spp. (Figures 2.12–2.13)

> Common name: Elephant skin disease (cattle).

Taxonomy: Protozoan (coccidia).

Geographic Distribution: *Besnoitia besnoiti* (cattle, goats) is found worldwide but is of greatest importance in Africa. *Besnoitia bennetti* (horses and donkeys) occurs primarily in Africa, southern Europe, and South America but is also found in North America.

Location in Host: Cysts are seen in the subcutaneous tissue and scleral conjunctiva of livestock.

Life Cycle: The definitive host of this coccidian parasite is the cat. Oocysts are shed in cat feces and are ingested by the intermediate host (cattle, horses, etc.). Parasites multiply in the endothelial cells and finally form large cysts in the subcutaneous tissue of intermediate hosts.

Laboratory Diagnosis: *Besnoitia* spp. often form cysts ("pearls") in the scleral conjunctiva that can easily be seen with the naked eye. Diagnosis can also be made by examining stained sections of skin biopsies for the presence of subcutaneous cysts.

Clinical Importance: Many cases are asymptomatic. However, an acute febrile illness can develop, followed by thickening and wrinkling of skin that makes the hide unsuitable for leather production. Affected animals may recover slowly. Although *Besnoitia* occurs in North America, its extent is unknown, and it rarely seems to cause clinical disease.

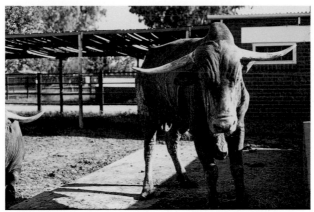

Fig. 2.12. Extensive skin thickening and wrinkling caused by *Besnoitia besnoiti*. This disease is most prevalent in Africa. Photo courtesy of Dr. Jeffrey F. Williams, Vanson HaloSource, Inc., Redmond, WA.

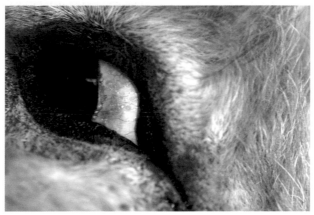

Fig. 2.13. Scleral "pearls," or cysts, of *Besnoitia bennetti* in the eye of a donkey in North America. Photo courtesy of Dr. Hany M. Elsheikha and Dr. Charles Mackenzie, College of Veterinary Medicine, Michigan State University, East Lansing, MI.

Detection of Parasites in the Blood

Various pathogenic and nonpathogenic protozoa and nematodes may be detected in blood samples from domestic animals. Most of these parasites are ingested by arthropod vectors during feeding and are present in the bloodstream of their mammalian hosts as a normal part of their life cycles.

IMMUNOLOGIC DETECTION OF BLOOD PARASITES

Although the focus of this book is the morphologic diagnosis of parasitism, it is important to recognize that immunologic tests are now widely used in conjunction with or in place of microscopic examination of blood smears for some blood-borne parasites and the use of these tests can be expected to increase in the future. Immunologic tests offer increased sensitivity compared to morphologic techniques in many cases and are especially valuable in some chronic hemoprotozoan infections and in canine and feline heartworm infection. In both cases, many infections are undetectable by routine microscopic tests. The commercial immunologic tests used most widely are the indirect fluorescent antibody test (IFA) and the enzyme-linked immunosorbent assay (ELISA).

Most commercial IFA tests detect the presence of parasite-specific antibody. Microscope slides or slide wells coated with parasites are incubated with serum from an animal suspected of infection. After washing, a second antibody specific for host immunoglobulin is added. The second antibody is conjugated with a compound (usually fluorescein) that will fluoresce when exposed to ultraviolet light. For example, an IFA test for canine *Babesia* infection is commonly used in North America. IFA tests require the use of a fluorescence microscope and cannot be performed in a veterinary practice.

ELISA tests can detect antibody to a parasite or parasite antigen, and some are available as kits that are useful in veterinary practices. In ELISA antibody tests the substrate is coated with parasite antigen. When the test blood sample is added, parasite-specific antibody will bind to the antigen. As in the IFA tests, a second host-specific antibody is then added and will bind to the antigen/antibody complexes on the substrate. The second antibody is conjugated to an enzyme, which is activated by the addition of the enzyme substrate and a detectable color change is produced. In ELISA tests for parasite antigen, the substrate of the test contains antibody specific for the parasite. When blood (or feces in the case of some parasitic infections) is added to the test, antibody will bind any parasite antigen present. This step is then followed by addition of the conjugated second antibody and enzyme substrate. In North America, ELISA tests for canine heartworm antigen have largely replaced morphologic examination of blood for the parasite.

MICROSCOPIC EXAMINATION OF BLOOD FOR PROTOZOAN PARASITES

Most hemoprotozoan parasites are intracellular in erythrocytes or white blood cells and may cause anemia. A routine thin blood smear is therefore useful both for assessing erythrocyte abnormalities and for detecting the presence of parasites. Parasites are most likely to be detected in blood smears during acute infection. Once infections become chronic, immunologic diagnostic techniques are usually more sensitive.

For microscopic examination of blood smears for hemoprotozoa, a Giemsa stain is most effective, but Wright's stain can also be used in most cases. Commercial stain kits used in many veterinary practices (an example is Dip Quick Stain, Jorgensen Laboratories, Loveland, CO, www.jorvet.com) will also stain hemoprotozoa when used as directed, but the stain will be of poorer quality. The following procedure can be followed when a Giemsa stain is used.

To prepare a thin blood smear place a drop of blood on one end of a microscope slide and draw the blood into a thin film as shown in Figure 3.1.

Giemsa Stain

1. Air-dry the blood film, protecting it from flies and other insects if it is not to be stained immediately.
2. Fix in absolute methanol for 5 minutes and air-dry.
3. Dilute stock Giemsa stain 1:20 with distilled water and flood the film (or place slide in staining jar). Fresh stain should be prepared at least every 2 days.
4. Stain for 30 minutes.

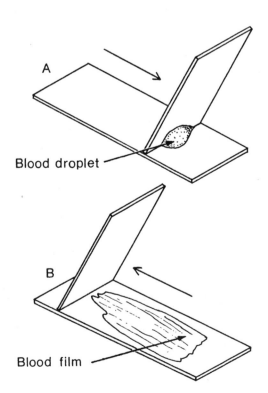

A

Blood droplet

B

Blood film

Fig. 3.1A and B. Technique for making a blood smear: (*A*) Bring a spreader slide back at an angle until it touches the drop of blood; wait until the drop flows laterally. (*B*) Draw the spreader slide away from the drop, maintaining an angle. The blood will spread into a smooth, thin film.

Table 3.1. Average diameters of erythrocytes

Animal	Erythrocyte Diameter (µm)
Horse	5.5
Cattle	5.8
Sheep	4.5
Goat	3.2
Dog	7.0
Cat	5.8
Chicken	7.0 × 12.0

Source: Measurements from Feldman et al. 2000.

5. Wash stain away gently with tap water.
6. Air-dry; parasite cytoplasm will stain blue, and nuclei will stain magenta.

The stained blood film can be scanned using the 40× objective of the microscope with use of the oil immersion lens for greater detail when suspected parasites are found.

The dimensions of blood parasites are best determined by means of an ocular micrometer (see Chap. 1). A micrometer is highly recommended for accurate measurement of parasites in blood and fecal samples. If a micrometer is not available, the size of the parasite on a blood film may be approximated by comparison with the dimensions of host erythrocytes (Table 3.1).

MICROSCOPIC EXAMINATION OF BLOOD FOR NEMATODE PARASITES

Many species of parasitic worms enter the bloodstream of the host to reach certain organs, where they develop to maturity. These parasites usually stay in the blood only minutes or hours; thus they are seldom seen in blood samples taken for diagnostic purposes. There are some filarial nematodes, however, whose larvae (microfilariae) are normally found in the peripheral blood. The microfilarial stage of these parasite species remains in the circulation until ingestion by the bloodsucking intermediate host. Microfilaria testing is most often performed for detection of canine heartworm infection, and the following discussion of techniques for microfilaria detection is directed specifically to heartworm testing. However, any species of microfilariae in the blood could be detected by the same microscopic techniques.

Although the techniques for microscopic detection of heartworm microfilariae are presented below, the ELISA adult-female antigen test for diagnosis of canine heartworm infection is the preferred screening test and has largely supplanted microfilaria tests in North America. Antigen tests are significantly more sensitive than microfilaria tests because many heartworm infections are amicrofilaremic. The absence of microfilariae may be due to low or single-sex worm burdens or immune clearance of microfilariae. Moreover, the macrolide heartworm preventatives are microfilaricidal and sterilize existing heartworm infections after several months of administration.

The American Heartworm Society currently recommends using an antigen test as the primary method of heartworm diagnosis. However, a microfilaria test (preferably in addition to an antigen test) must also be performed annually on any dog receiving diethylcarbamazine (DEC) prophylaxis because of the serious reactions that may follow treatment of microfilaremic dogs with DEC. Any dog testing positive on an antigen test should also be tested for microfilariae, both to validate the antigen test and to determine if microfilaricidal treatment is necessary. If a microfilaria test is used alone for heartworm testing, one of the concentration techniques (Knott's or filter test) must be used.

Antigen tests currently available in the USA are available in ELISA, immunochromatographic, and hemagglutination formats. Although differences in sensitivity among these tests have been found experimentally, they are not statistically significant. False-negative results are uncommon and are usually the result of lab error, although a small number (<1%) of antigen-negative dogs will be microfilaremic. Available tests are also highly specific; however, the hemagglutination test may produce false-positive results if red cell sedimentation is confused with agglutination.

Diagnosis of heartworm infection in cats is more difficult than in dogs. Several of the antigen tests can be used in cats, but they often produce false-negative results because of the low worm burdens usually found in cats. Similarly, cats are rarely microfilaremic and may develop disease before the adult stage, detectable by antigen testing, is present. To improve the sensitivity of heartworm detection in cats, heartworm antibody tests have been developed. These tests can detect infection earlier than antigen tests but may only indicate exposure to the parasite rather than active infection. Care should be taken in interpreting a feline antibody test, and the results of that test alone should not be used to establish a diagnosis of heartworm infection. In a cat showing clinical signs consistent with heartworm infection, both antigen and antibody tests should be performed as part of the diagnostic workup.

For current recommendations of the American Heartworm Society relating to diagnosis and treatment of heartworm infection in dogs and cats, consult the American Heartworm Society Website: www.heartwormsociety.org.

Tests for Canine Heartworm Microfilariae in Blood Samples

The following techniques can be used to detect microfilariae in blood samples. The canine heartworm, *Dirofilaria immitis*, is found throughout the world. In North America, dogs may also be infected with *Dipetalonema* (= *Acanthocheilonema*) *reconditum* or, rarely, with *Dirofilaria striata,* a parasite of wild felids in North and South America. In parts of Europe, Asia, and Africa *Dirofilaria repens* parasitizes dogs. When a microfilaria test is used for heartworm diagnosis, the microfilariae of other species must be differentiated from those of *D. immitis*.

Microfilariae of *Dirofilaria immitis* can be reliably differentiated from those of *D. striata* and *Dipetalonema reconditum* based on size (Table 3.2) measured with an eyepiece micrometer (see Chap. 1 for micrometer calibration procedure). Other criteria can also be used to discriminate between the two species, but they are less dependable. Determination of the length, width, and shape of the head of a microfilaria should allow identification of almost all canine microfilariae in North America. The standard measurements of these microfilariae were determined on 2% formalin-fixed specimens; use of other fixatives or lysing solutions may alter the size of the organisms. Similarly, storage of whole blood for more than 3 days may cause some *D. immitis* microfilariae to shrink in length to the size of *D. reconditum*.

Table 3.2. Distinguishing characteristics of *Dirofilaria immitis, Dirofilaria striata,* and *Dipetalonema reconditum* microfilariae (fixed in 2% formalin)

Distinguishing Feature	*Dirofilaria immitis*	*Dirofilaria striata*	*Dipetalonema reconditum*
Size (μm)			
Width	5–7.5	5–6	4.5–5.5
Length	295–325	360–385	250–288
Head	Tapered	Tapered	Blunt
Tail	Straight	Curved	Buttonhook (30%) or curved
Body shape	Straight	S-shaped	Curved
Motion	Stationary	Stationary	Progressive
Relative number	Few to many	Few	Few

Direct Smear

The direct smear is the simplest and most rapid of the procedures to be described for microfilariae. It is not a very sensitive technique but can be used in conjunction with an adult heartworm antigen test to determine if microfilariae are present or to evaluate the pattern of movement of microfilariae when attempting to differentiate between *Dirofilaria* and *Dipetalonema*.

1. Place one drop of venous blood onto a clean microscope slide and coverslip.
2. Examine the coverslip area under low magnification (10×) of the microscope. Look for undulating movements of larvae, which may retain motility for as long as 24 hours.

Hematocrit Test

This technique is only slightly more sensitive than the direct smear.

1. Draw fresh whole blood into a microhematocrit tube.
2. Spin for 3 minutes in a hematocrit tube centrifuge.
3. Examine the plasma portion of the separated blood, while still in the tube, under low magnification (10×). Moving microfilariae will be present in the plasma above the buffy coat.

The direct smear and microhematocrit techniques may not detect infections with only small numbers of microfilariae. Therefore, if a microfilariae test is used as a screening procedure for heartworm infection, one of the following concentration techniques is preferred.

Modified Knott's Test

The Modified Knott's technique is the preferred concentration method for the detection and identification of microfilariae in blood.

1. Draw a sample of blood into a syringe containing anticoagulant such as EDTA or heparin.
2. Mix 1 ml of the blood with 9 ml of a 2% formalin solution. If not well mixed, the red cells will not be thoroughly lysed by the hypotonic formalin solution, making the test much more difficult to read. Microfilariae, but not red cells, will be fixed by 2% formalin. If 10% formalin is used (the concentration used for fixation of tissues), red cells will also be fixed and not lysed.
3. Centrifuge the mixture at 1200 rpm for 5 minutes (or as for fecal flotation procedures) and discard the supernatant.
4. Add 1 drop of 0.1% methylene blue to the sediment, mix well, and transfer the stained sediment to a microscope slide using a Pasteur pipette to collect the entire sample.
5. Examine using the 10× microscope objective. Microfilariae will be fixed in an extended position with nuclei stained blue.

An alternative procedure using the same amount of blood is the filter test, which traps microfilariae on a filter that is examined with the microscope. This technique can be performed more quickly than the Modified Knott's Test, but microfilariae are not easily measured for identification.

Filter Test

Kits containing filter apparatus, filters, lysing solution, and stain are commercially available (Difil-Test®, EVSCO Pharmaceuticals, Buena, NJ 08310). Components of the test can also be purchased. Use of 2% formalin as the lysing solution is recommended, since other lysing solutions may cause significant changes in the size of microfilariae.

1. Mix 1 ml of blood with 9 ml lysing solution in a syringe.
2. Attach the syringe to the filter holder containing a filter with a 5 μm pore size and empty the syringe.
3. Refill syringe with water and pass it through the filter to wash away remaining small debris.
4. Refill syringe with air, reattach to the filter apparatus, and express.
5. Unscrew the filter assembly, remove the filter with forceps, and place the filter on a microscope slide.
6. Add 1 drop of 0.1% methylene blue, coverslip, and examine at 10×.

BLOOD PARASITES OF DOGS AND CATS

PARASITE: *Babesia canis* and *B. gibsoni* (Figures 3.2–3.3)

Taxonomy: Protozoan (piroplasm). *Babesia gibsoni* consists of more than one genetically distinct but morphologically identical species.

Geographic Distribution: *Babesia* mostly occurs in the tropical and subtropical regions of the world. *Babesia canis* is worldwide in distribution; in the USA, it occurs in the southeast. *Babesia gibsoni* infects canids in North Africa and the Far East and has recently been reported in various states in the USA.

Location in Host: Canine red blood cells. *Babesia* spp. have been described in cats but are not widely distributed and do not appear to be present in North America.

Life Cycle: In North America, dogs acquire *B. canis* and *B. gibsoni* infections from the brown dog tick, *Rhipicephalus sanguineus*. Other tick vectors include *Dermacentor reticulatus* in Europe and *Haemaphysalis leachi* in Africa.

Laboratory Diagnosis: Piroplasms can be detected in erythrocytes on Wright- or Giemsa-stained blood smears. Serologic tests (IFA) can also be used and are a more sensitive diagnostic technique in chronic infections. *Babesia canis* is pear shaped and usually occurs in pairs; *B. gibsoni* is round to oval shaped.

Size:	*B. canis*	4–5 μm
	B. gibsoni	1–3 μm

Clinical Importance: Severity of clinical disease may range from mild to life-threatening. Anemia, hemolytic crisis, and multi-organ failure can occur. North American and European strains appear to be less pathogenic than those infecting dogs in Africa and Asia.

PARASITE: *Hepatozoon* spp. (Figure 3.4)

Taxonomy: Protozoan (hemogregarine).

Geographic Distribution: *Hepatozoon canis* occurs worldwide, while the distribution of *H. americanum* appears to be limited to the southeastern USA.

Location in Host: Gamonts are found in polymorphonuclear leukocytes (*H. americanum, H. canis*) and meronts in skeletal muscle (*H. americanum*) or various organs (*H. canis*) of dogs, cats, and various wild carnivores.

Life Cycle: The tick intermediate host acquires infection during feeding. Dogs become infected by ingesting infected ticks. *Hepatozoon americanum* is transmitted by *Amblyomma maculatum* (the Gulf Coast tick), and the vector of *H. canis* is *Rhipicephalus sanguineus* (the brown dog tick).

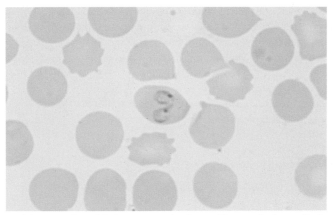

Fig. 3.2. Erythrocyte containing pear-shaped *Babesia canis* piroplasms. The parasite is usually found in pairs, as many as eight piroplasms may be found in a single red blood cell.

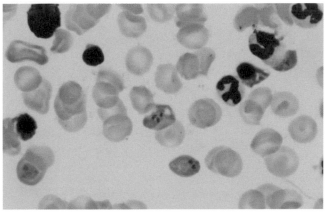

Fig. 3.3. *Babesia gibsoni* is a smaller organism than *B. canis*. The pear shape seen so clearly with *B. canis* is much less distinct with *B. gibsoni*.

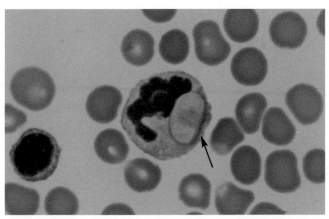

Fig. 3.4. *Hepatozoon* gamont in a polymorphonucleocyte. The parasite is sausage shaped with a centrally compact nucleus that stains only faintly in this specimen (*arrow*). *Hepatozoon americanum* is rarely present in blood films, and muscle biopsies are more commonly used for diagnosis.

Laboratory Diagnosis: Sausage-shaped *Hepatozoon* gamonts can be detected in polymorphonuclear leukocytes in Wright- or Geimsa-stained blood smears. Although this method of diagnosis can be used for *H. canis, H. americanum* is rarely found on blood smears. Diagnosis of this species generally occurs by the detection of meronts in skeletal muscle biopsies or on histopathology after necropsy.

Size: gamonts 8–12 μm × 3–6 μm

Clinical Importance: *Hepatozoon americanum* can cause severe disease, with fever, depression, joint pain, myositis, periosteal bone proliferation, and chronic wasting. *Hepatozoon canis* infections are usually subclinical.

PARASITE: ***Cytauxzoon felis*** (Figure 3.5)

Taxonomy: Protozoan (piroplasm).

Geographic Distribution: Southern USA.

Location in Host: Merozoites occur in red blood cells, and schizonts occur in histiocytes of bobcats and cats.

Life Cycle: Infection transmission occurs through the blood-feeding activities of the tick vectors. *Dermacentor variabilis* has been used to transmit infections experimentally.

Laboratory Diagnosis: Merozoites are detected in red blood cells (1–4 merozoites/erythrocyte) in Wright- or Giemsa-stained blood smears. Schizonts are detected in mononuclear cells in bone-marrow aspirates.

Size: 1–2 μm

Clinical Importance: *Cytauxzoon felis* is highly pathogenic in cats. Infections are usually fatal; cats die within a few days of the onset of clinical signs. Anemia, depression, high fever, icterus, hepatomegaly, and splenomegaly occur.

PARASITE: ***Leishmania*** spp. (Figures 3.6–3.7)
          Common name: Visceral and cutaneous leishmaniasis.

Taxonomy: Protozoan (hemoflagellate). Species include *L. donovani, L. tropica, L. infantum, L. chagasi, L. braziliensis, L. mexicana.*

Geographic Distribution: Worldwide.

Location in Host: Amastigotes occur in macrophages and cells of the reticuloendothelial system of various organs (skin, spleen, liver, bone marrow, lymph nodes).

Life Cycle: Blood-feeding sand flies (*Lutzomyia, Phlebotomus*) serve as intermediate hosts.

Laboratory Diagnosis: Diagnosis occurs by detection of amastigotes in macrophages in stained smears made from needle aspirate biopsies of lymph node, bone marrow, or spleen or in impression smears of skin lesions. Amastigotes are rarely seen in stained peripheral-blood smears. Serological and PCR techniques are also used in diagnosis.

Size: 2.5–5.0 × 1.5–2.0 μm

Clinical Importance: Infection in dogs is often subclinical. However, disease may develop involving various visceral organs and skin, resulting in cutaneous lesions, lethargy, progressive weight loss, and anorexia that may end in death. Infection with *L. infantum* has recently been found to be widespread in foxhounds in the USA. Cats are rarely infected. Leishmaniasis is a serious, potentially fatal disease in humans. Dogs serve as an important reservoir host of the parasite in some parts of the world.

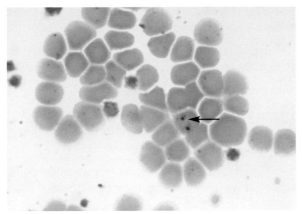

Fig. 3.5. Small *Cytauxzoon felis* merozoites in infected erythrocytes (*arrow*) have a dark nucleus and a light blue cytoplasm on Wright- or Giemsa-stained blood smears. Photo courtesy of Dr. Karen Snowden, College of Veterinary Medicine, Texas A&M University, College Station, TX.

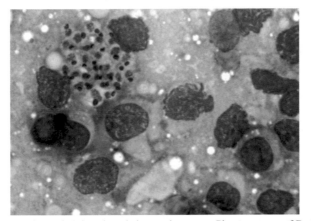

Fig. 3.6. *Leishmania* spp. amastigotes in a lymph node impression smear. Photo courtesy of Dr. Karen Snowden, College of Veterinary Medicine, Texas A&M University, College Station, TX.

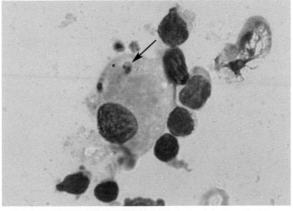

Fig. 3.7. *Leishmania* amastigote (*arrow*) in a macrophage from a canine lymph node. The small round kinetoplast can be seen adjacent to the nucleus in this amastigote. Photo courtesy of Dr. Bernard Feldman, Virginia-Maryland Regional College of Veterinary Medicine, Virginia Tech, Blacksburg, VA.

169

PARASITE: *Trypanosoma cruzi* (Figure 3.8)
                 Common name: Chagas Disease.

Taxonomy: Protozoan (hemoflagellate). Dogs and cats can also be infected with *T. brucei, T. congolense,* and *T. evansi,* trypanosome species more commonly associated with large animals (see below).

Geographic Distribution: North and South America.

Location in Host: Trypomastigotes occur in the blood; amastigotes and epimastigotes occur in skeletal muscle, reticuloendothelial cells, and various other tissues of humans, dogs, cats, and many wildlife mammalian species.

Life Cycle: Triatomids (kissing or assassin bugs) pass trypomastigotes in the feces during blood feeding on the vertebrate definitive host. Parasites enter the definitive host through mucous membranes or through the triatomid bite-wound site.

Laboratory Diagnosis: Trypomastigotes are detected on Wright- or Giemsa-stained blood smears early in infection. Diagnosis in chronic or light infections may require serological tests, culture, or xenodiagnosis.

   Size: 16–20 µm

Clinical Importance: Infection with *T. cruzi* is highly pathogenic, causing acute and chronic cardiac disease. Lymphadenopathy, pale mucous membranes, lethargy, ascites, hepatomegaly, splenomegaly, anorexia, diarrhea, and neurologic signs may be seen. Infection in dogs and cats is relatively uncommon in North America.

PARASITE: *Dirofilaria immitis* (Figures 3.9–3.10)
                 Common name: Heartworm.

Taxonomy: Nematode (order Spirurida).

Geographic Distribution: Worldwide. *Dirofilaria repens* is a largely nonpathogenic parasite of the subcutaneous tissue in Mediterranean countries, Africa, and Egypt, and *D. striata* is a rare parasite of dogs in the southeastern USA.

Location in Host: Adult worms are found in the pulmonary arteries and right ventricle of dogs, wild canids, and ferrets. Cats are much less likely than dogs to become infected, and feline infections are rarely patent.

Life Cycle: Mosquitoes serve as intermediate hosts, acquiring microfilariae and transmitting infective third-stage larvae while blood feeding. The prepatent period in dogs is about 6 months.

Laboratory Diagnosis: The most sensitive technique for heartworm diagnosis is detection of antigen using one of the various commercial antigen kits for use with serum, plasma, and/or whole blood. Less sensitive is testing for microfilariae in blood samples using a filter test or the Knott's Test, which are equal in ability to detect microfilariae. However, the Knott's Test should be used for specific identification of microfilariae (on the basis of size and morphology).

   Size: 295–325 µm × 5–7.5 µm

Clinical Importance: Heartworm infection is highly pathogenic and is an important medical health issue in both canine and feline medicine. Chronic heartworm infection in dogs can lead to fatal right-sided congestive heart failure. A liver failure (or Caval) syndrome occurs in some dogs with heavy worm burdens (>100) that, without treatment, leads to a rapidly fatal hemolytic crisis. Heartworm infection in cats can be subclinical or result in serious chronic disease (respiratory or vomiting/gastrointestinal) or cats may die acutely.

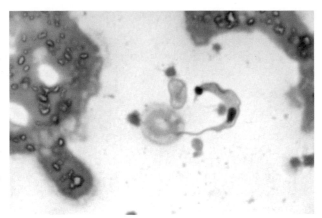

Fig. 3.8. Stained trypomastigotes of *Trypanosoma cruzi* in a blood smear from an infected dog. The organisms often assume a C shape in blood smears. The dark-staining kinetoplast can easily be seen in this specimen. Photo courtesy of Dr. Karen Snowden, College of Veterinary Medicine, Texas A&M University, College Station, TX.

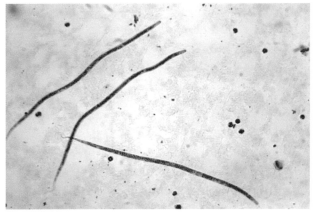

Fig. 3.9. Microfilariae of *Dirofilaria immitis* recovered from a blood sample using the Modified Knott's technique. Heartworm microfilariae have gently tapered heads and relatively straight tails. Photo courtesy of Dr. Thomas Nolan, School of Veterinary Medicine, University of Pennsylvania, Philadelphia, PA.

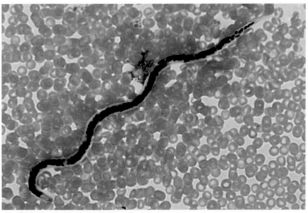

Fig. 3.10. Microfilariae are at an earlier developmental stage than first-stage larvae and do not contain a digestive tract. Only dark-staining cell nuclei can be seen in this *D. immitis* microfilaria. Photo courtesy of Dr. Dwight Bowman, College of Veterinary Medicine, Cornell University, Ithaca, NY.

171

PARASITE: *Dipetalonema* (=*Acanthocheilonema*) *reconditum* (Figures 3.11–3.12)

Taxonomy: Nematode (order Spirurida). The genus *Dipetalonema* has been revised in recent years and the correct name for *D. reconditum* is now considered to be *Acanthocheilonema reconditum*. However, this name is not widely used in veterinary medicine. To avoid confusion, the older name, *Dipetalonema,* is used here.

Geographic Distribution: USA, South America, Africa, southern Europe, Asia.

Location in Host: Subcutaneous tissues of dogs and various wild canids.

Life Cycle: Dogs acquire infections from fleas (*Ctenocephalides, Pulex*) and lice (*Linognathus, Heterodoxus*). Arthropods ingest microfilariae in the blood (*Ctenocephalides, Pulex, Linognathus*) or skin (*Heterodoxus*) of infected canids.

Laboratory Diagnosis: Diagnosis is by detection of microfilariae as for *D. immitis*. Canine heartworm antigen tests do not give a positive reaction in the presence of *Dipetalonema* infection. *Dipetalonema reconditum* microfilariae have a blunt anterior end, and the tails of some individuals may form a small hook or U shape, usually referred to as a "buttonhook."

Size: 250–288 μm × 4.5–5.5 μm

Clinical Importance: Infections with *D. reconditum* are subclinical. The accurate diagnosis of *D. reconditum* infections in dogs is important in order to prevent misdiagnoses of heartworm infection.

BLOOD PARASITES OF LIVESTOCK AND HORSES

PARASITE: *Babesia* **spp.** (Figure 3.13)
              Common name: Redwater, Texas fever, tick fever.

Taxonomy: Protozoan (piroplasm).

Geographic Distribution: Worldwide, particularly in tropical regions.

Location in Host: Red blood cells of cattle (at least six species, including *B. bovis, B. divergens, B. bigemina, B. major*) and sheep and goats (*B. motasi, B. ovis*).

Life Cycle: A variety of tick genera, including *Boophilus, Ixodes,* and *Rhipicephalus,* act as intermediate hosts of *Babesia* spp. Ticks acquire the parasite during feeding.

Laboratory Diagnosis: In acute infection, blood smears stained with Giemsa or Wright's stain can be examined for parasites in red blood cells. In chronic infection parasites are difficult to find in peripheral blood, and therefore antibody tests, including IFA and ELISA tests, are used for diagnosis. *Babesia* typically appears as pairs of organisms in red blood cells, although erythrocytes may also contain single organisms.

Size: 1.5–4.5 μm × 0.4–2.0 μm, depending on species (*B. bigemina:* 4.5 μm × 2.5 μm; *B. bovis:* 2.4 μm × 1.5 μm)

Clinical Importance: In susceptible animals infection can lead to the development of anemia, hemoglobinuria, and fever, with death often occurring during the acute phase of infection. Unlike many parasitic diseases, young animals are less likely to develop disease than adults. Bovine babesiosis has been eradicated from the USA.

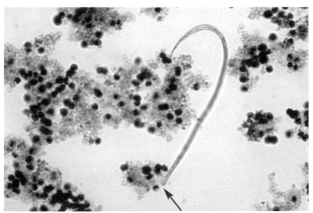

Fig. 3.11. Microfilariae of *Dipetalonema* (= *Acanthocheilonema*) *reconditum* in a Modified Knott's Test. The anterior end (*arrow*) is blunter than that of *D. immitis*. Photo courtesy of Dr. Thomas Nolan, School of Veterinary Medicine, University of Pennsylvania, Philadelphia, PA.

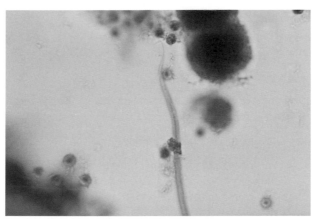

Fig. 3.12. The tails of some microfilariae of *Dipetalonema* form a buttonhook shape when fixed. Microfilariae of *D. reconditum* are smaller than those of *D. immitis*. See Table 3.2 for a comparison of morphologic characteristics of microfilariae found in dogs in North America. Photo courtesy of Dr. Jeffrey F. Williams, Vanson HaloSource, Inc., Redmond, WA.

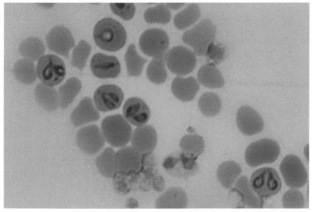

Fig. 3.13. *Babesia bigemina* can be seen in this bovine blood smear. The teardrop-shaped organisms are present in pairs in several erythrocytes. *Babesia trautmanni*, a cause of porcine babesiosis in parts of Europe and Africa, has a similar morphology. Photo courtesy of Dr. Alvin Gajadhar, Centre for Animal Parasitology, CFIA, Saskatoon, Saskatchewan, Canada.

PARASITE: *Babesia equi, B. caballi* (Figure 3.14)

Taxonomy: Protozoan (piroplasm).

Geographic Distribution: Equine babesiosis is endemic in Central and South America, Africa, southern Europe, the Middle East, and parts of Asia.

Location in Host: Equine erythrocytes. Tick intermediate hosts include species of *Rhipicephalus, Hyalomma,* and *Dermacentor.*

Life Cycle: Similar to ruminant *Babesia* spp.

Laboratory Diagnosis: Blood smears are examined in acute infection. Chronic carriers are unlikely to show parasites in the peripheral blood. ELISA and IFA tests are used for detecting antibody to parasites in chronic infection.

Size:	*B. equi*	2 μm
	B. caballi	2.5–4 μm

Clinical Importance: Equine babesiosis can cause anemia, hemoglobinuria, and edema. *Babesia caballi* may cause incoordination and paralysis.

PARASITE: *Theileria* **spp.** (Figures 3.15–3.16)
Common name: East Coast fever, corridor disease, African Coast fever.

Taxonomy: Protozoan (piroplasm).

Geographic Distribution: Species of greatest importance are *T. parva* in East Central and South Africa and *T. annulata* in North Africa and southern Europe.

Location in Host: Bovine erythrocytes and lymph nodes.

Life Cycle: *Rhipicephalus* (*T. parva*) and *Hyalomma* (*T. annulata*) ticks are infected when they ingest host red blood cells. Following development in the tick, sporozoites are passed to cattle during feeding and enter lymphocytes, where schizogony occurs, releasing merozoites that infect red blood cells.

Laboratory Diagnosis: Schizonts can be seen in smears of lymph-node biopsies and, in the case of *T. annulata*, infection may be diagnosed by finding infected red blood cells in a blood smear. *Theileria parva* is unlikely to be present in blood smears except in advanced cases. IFA and ELISA tests are available, but because of the acute nature of clinical disease, these tests are of greater use in assessing host response in recovered animals.

Size:	piroplasms in red blood cells	1.5–2.0 μm × 0.5–1.0 μm
	schizonts in lymphocytes	approx. 8 μm

Clinical Importance: Susceptible animals develop fever, lymphadenopathy, depression, and nasal discharge; there is high mortality in nonimmune animals. Chronic disease is associated with a variety of symptoms, including diarrhea and reduced production.

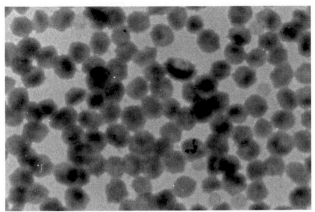

Fig. 3.14. Blood smear containing *Babesia equi* in equine erythrocytes. Both equine *Babesia* spp. are often seen in pairs in red blood cells. In addition, *Babesia equi* may undergo a further division and produce four organisms in the form of a cross, the so-called "Maltese cross." Photo courtesy of Dr. Alvin Gajadhar, Centre for Animal Parasitology, CFIA, Saskatoon, Saskatchewan, Canada.

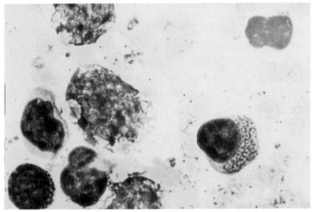

Fig. 3.15. *Theileria parva* multinucleated schizont in a lymphocyte. The species of *Theileria* are difficult to differentiate morphologically. Photo courtesy of Dr. Andrew Peregrine, Ontario Veterinary College, University of Guelph, Guelph, Ontario, Canada.

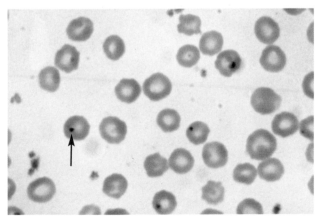

Fig. 3.16. *Theileria* sp. erythrocytic forms in a blood smear (*arrow*). Photo courtesy of Dr. Karen Snowden, College of Veterinary Medicine, Texas A&M University, College Station, TX.

Parasite: *Trypanosoma* **spp.** (Figures 3.17–3.22)

   Common name: Nagana, sleeping sickness, surra, dourine.

Taxonomy: Protozoan (flagellate).

Geographic Distribution: Clinically important livestock species, including *T. congolense, T. brucei brucei, T. simiae, T. vivax,* and *T. evansi,* are all found in Africa. *Trypanosoma evansi* and *T. vivax* are also found in South America and parts of Asia. *Trypanosoma theileri* (cattle only) and *T. melophagium* (sheep only) occur worldwide. Another species, *T. equiperdum* (horses), is found in tropical and subtropical regions.

Location in Host: Bloodstream of ruminants, horses, swine, and other domestic animals. *Trypanosoma brucei* can also be found in other tissues, including the heart and central nervous system. *Trypanosoma equiperdum* is found in the urethra of stallions and vagina of mares.

Life Cycle: Trypanosomes are transmitted to the host by biting flies. The intermediate host of *T. congolense, T. vivax, T. brucei,* and *T. simiae* is the tsetse fly (*Glossina*) in Africa. In other areas tabanid and other biting flies transmit *T. vivax* and *T. evansi.* Tabanid flies are also the intermediate host of *T. theileri* in cattle, while the sheep ked (*Melophagus ovinus*) is the intermediate host of *T. melophagium.* The exception to fly transmission is *T. equiperdum,* which is transmitted venereally.

Laboratory Diagnosis: In acute infection most trypanosome species can usually be detected in wet mounts of blood. Species of trypanosomes can be differentiated based on size, presence or absence of a free flagellum, location and size of the kinetoplast, and characteristics of the undulating membrane. An ELISA antigen test and DNA probes have been developed for detection of African trypanosomiasis in cattle. *Trypanosoma equiperdum* infection is diagnosed by a complement fixation test.

Size:		
	T. vivax	20–26 μm
	T. brucei	12–35 μm
	T. congolense	9–18 μm
	T. evansi	15–35 μm
	T. theileri	60–70 μm, may be up to 120 μm
	T. melophagium	50–60 μm
	T. simiae	13–18 μm

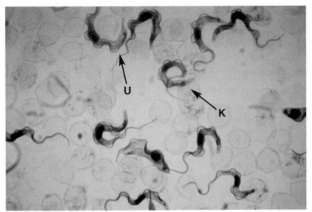

Fig. 3.17. *Trypanosoma brucei* and *T. congolense* are found in domestic mammals in Africa. *Trypanosoma brucei* has a prominent undulating membrane (U) and a kinetoplast that is located subterminally (K). Photo courtesy of Dr. Andrew Peregrine, Ontario Veterinary College, University of Guelph, Guelph, Ontario, Canada.

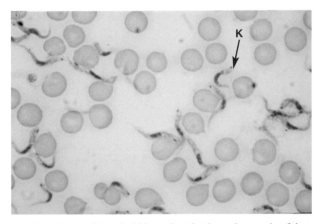

Fig. 3.18. *Trypanosoma congolense* has a subterminal kinetoplast that is on the margin of the trypanosome (K). Its undulating membrane is not distinctive. Photo courtesy of Dr. Andrew Peregrine, Ontario Veterinary College, University of Guelph, Guelph, Ontario, Canada.

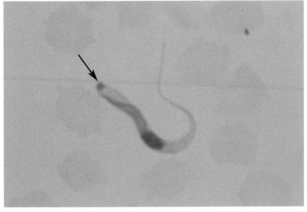

Fig. 3.19. *Trypanosoma vivax* is found in Africa and other parts of the world. Its kinetoplast is at the end of the organism (*arrow*), and its undulating membrane is not distinctive. Photo courtesy of Dr. Andrew Peregrine, Ontario Veterinary College, University of Guelph, Guelph, Ontario, Canada.

Clinical Importance: The principal clinical signs of trypanosomiasis are anemia accompanied by fever, edema, and loss of condition. Mortality may be high, especially if other disease agents are also present. *Trypanosoma equiperdum* produces the disease known as dourine in horses, which is marked by genital and ventral edema, abortion, nervous system disease, and emaciation. *Trypanosoma melophagium* and *T. theileri* are widespread nonpathogenic species that may occasionally be seen in blood smears.

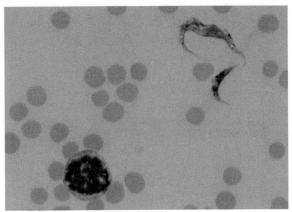

Fig. 3.20. *Trypanosoma theileri* is found worldwide in cattle, and a similar parasite, *T. melophagium,* occurs in sheep. Parasites are occasionally seen in blood smears but rarely are of clinical importance. These species can be distinguished from the pathogenic trypanosome species by their large size (50 μm or more). This blood smear from a calf demonstrates the size variation that can occur with *T. theileri.*

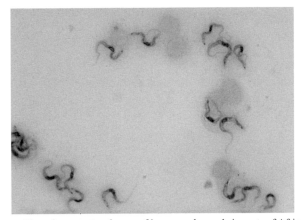

Fig. 3.21. *Trypanosoma evansi* is an important pathogen of horses and camels in parts of Africa, Asia, and Latin America. It is difficult to distinguish from *T. brucei* microscopically. Photo courtesy of Dr. Jeffrey F. Williams, Vanson HaloSource, Inc., Redmond, WA.

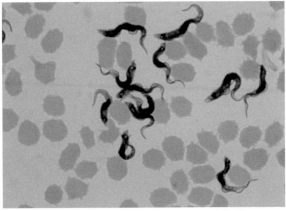

Fig. 3.22. *Trypanosoma simiae* is a parasite of African warthogs that is transmitted by the tsetse fly to domestic pigs and camels. Swine may also be infected with other trypanosome species. Photo courtesy of Dr. Andrew Peregrine, Ontario Veterinary College, University of Guelph, Guelph, Ontario, Canada.

PARASITE: *Setaria* spp. (Figure 3.23)

Taxonomy: Nematode (order Spirurida).

Geographic Distribution: Worldwide.

Location in Host: Adult worms are found primarily in the peritoneal cavity of ruminants and equids.

Life Cycle: Microfilariae in the blood are ingested by mosquitoes. The infective third larval stage develops in the mosquito; transmission to the definitive host occurs during feeding.

Laboratory Diagnosis: Detection of sheathed microfilariae in blood smears.

    Size: approx. 200–300 µm in length

Clinical Importance: *Setaria* has no clinical importance, with the exception of rare cases of abnormal migration of parasites in the nervous system.

BLOOD PARASITES OF BIRDS

PARASITE: *Leucocytozoon* spp. (Figures 3.24–3.25)

Taxonomy: Protozoan (hemosporozoa).

Geographic Distribution: Important species include *L. simondi,* which is found worldwide in domestic and wild ducks and geese; *L. smithi* in North American and European domestic and wild turkeys; and *L. caulleryi* in chickens in Asia.

Location in Host: Gamonts (microgamonts and macrogamonts) occur in leukocytes and erythrocytes.

Life Cycle: Black flies (*Simulium* spp. and other simulids) transmit infections to birds during blood feeding.

Laboratory Diagnosis: Gamonts are detected in white and red blood cells on Wright- or Giemsa-stained blood smears. Meronts are detected in stained tissue sections.

    Size: gamonts 14–22 µm

Clinical Importance: *Leucocytozoon* is pathogenic in ducks, geese, and turkeys, especially in younger birds. Clinical signs vary somewhat with species but can include lethargy, emaciation, and acute or chronic fatalities.

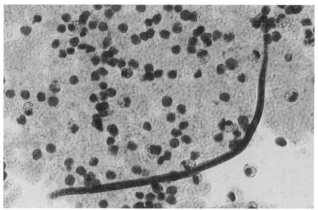

Fig. 3.23. Microfilariae of *Setaria* spp. may occasionally be seen in ruminant or equine blood samples but have no clinical significance. A clear sheath can often be seen projecting beyond the end of the larva, although it is not evident in this specimen. Photo courtesy of Dr. Jeffrey F. Williams, Vanson HaloSource, Inc., Redmond, WA.

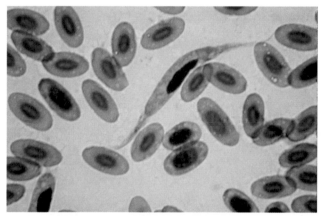

Fig. 3.24. Host leukocytes and erythrocytes containing the sausage-shaped *Leucocytozoon* gamonts appear elongated, with the remnants of the nucleus pushed to one side and the cytoplasm extending beyond the parasite and forming "horns." Photo courtesy of Dr. David Baker, School of Veterinary Medicine, Louisiana State University, Baton Rouge, LA.

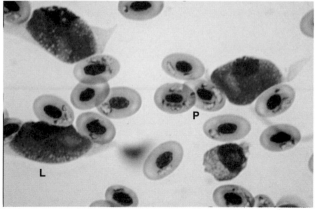

Fig. 3.25. Birds may be infected with more than one species of protozoan. Both *Leucocytozoon* (L) and *Plasmodium* (P) are present in this hawk. Photo courtesy of Dr. David Baker, School of Veterinary Medicine, Louisiana State University, Baton Rouge, LA.

PARASITE: *Haemoproteus* **spp.** (Figure 3.26)

Taxonomy: Protozoan (hemosporozoa).

Geographic Distribution: Worldwide (except *H. meleagridis,* which occurs only in North America).

Location in Host: Gamonts (microgamonts and macrogamonts) occur in erythrocytes of pigeons and doves (*H. columbae, H. sacharovi*), wild and domestic turkeys (*H. meleagridis*), and wild and domestic ducks and geese (*H. nettionis*).

Life Cycle: Birds acquire infections from blood-feeding hippoboscid flies, midges (*Culicoides*), and deer flies (*Chrysops* spp.), which act as intermediate hosts.

Laboratory Diagnosis: Gamonts are detected in red blood cells on Wright- or Giemsa-stained blood smears. The gamonts of *Haemoproteus* may vary in size and contain pigment granules. They appear morphologically identical to those of *Plasmodium* spp.

Size: approx. 7 μm

Clinical Importance: Infections are usually subclinical.

PARASITE: *Plasmodium* **spp.** (Figure 3.27, 3.25)
Common name: Malaria.

Taxonomy: Protozoan (hemosporozoa).

Geographic Distribution: Worldwide.

Location in Host: Erythrocytes and various other tissues in a wide variety of birds.

Life Cycle: Mosquitoes act as the intermediate host for *Plasmodium.* The parasite is transmitted during insect feeding.

Laboratory Diagnosis: Gamonts, merozoites, and meronts are detected in red blood cells on Wright- or Giemsa-stained blood smears. Gamonts of *Plasmodium* appear morphologically identical to those of *Haemoproteus* spp.

Size: gamonts 7–8 μm

Clinical Importance: Most species are nonpathogenic. Exceptions are *P. cathemerium* and *P. matutinum* in canaries; *P. gallinaceum* and *P. juxtanucleare* in chickens; *P. hermani* in turkeys; and *P. relictum* in pigeons. Birds infected with these species may become anemic, with high fatality rates possible.

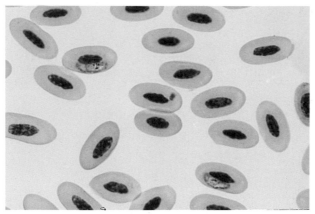

Fig. 3.26. Gamonts of *Haemoproteus* in a Swainson's hawk. The gamonts are often crescent shaped and wrapped around the nucleus of the host erythrocyte. Pigment granules can be seen inside the gamont. Photo courtesy of Dr. Robert Ridley, College of Veterinary Medicine, Kansas State University, Manhattan, KS.

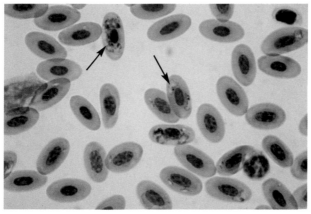

Fig 3.27. The appearance of multiple stages of the parasite (signet-ring stage, meronts, and gamonts) in infected erythrocytes differentiates *Plasmodium* infection from *Haemoproteus* (in which only gamonts are found). In this sample from a cockatoo, several stages of the parasite are present (*arrows*). Photo courtesy of Dr. David Baker, School of Veterinary Medicine, Louisiana State University, Baton Rouge, LA.

Diagnosis of Arthropod Parasites

Ellis C. Greiner, University of Florida, contributing author

The phylum Arthropoda contains many species that parasitize domestic and wild animals and humans. The most familiar of these parasites are ticks, mites (class Arachnida, subclass Acari), and insects (class Insecta). Aquatic animals are parasitized by many crustaceans that also belong to this phylum (see Chap. 5). All arthropods have jointed appendages and exoskeletons. The organisms pictured in this chapter represent a selection of arthropods that are common or important in domestic animals.

SUBCLASS ACARI (MITES AND TICKS)

The bodies of mites and ticks are divided into two parts: the gnathosoma, which contains the mouthparts on a false head (basis capitulum), and the idiosoma, which comprises the remainder of the animal and to which the legs are attached. After hatching from the egg, mites and ticks pass through larval and nymphal stages before becoming adults. Larvae of ticks and mites have six legs; while nymphs and adults have eight legs. Nymphal ticks and mites usually closely resemble the adults but are smaller and lack a genital opening.

Mite Identification

Parasitic mites are usually microscopic, rarely exceeding 1 mm in length. Female mites are usually larger than males. Mites are covered by a relatively soft integument through which the smaller forms respire. The larger forms breathe through openings called stigmata, sometimes used in identification. Scales, spines, or setae (hairs) on the body and claws or suckers on the legs (Fig. 4.1) are used in identifying the organisms. Many common mange, itch, and scab mites resemble one another, but can be differentiated on the basis of the characteristics outlined in Table 4.1.

Most common mite infestations are diagnosed by deep or superficial skin scrapings. For a deep skin scraping, a dulled, rounded scalpel blade (#10) and the area of skin to be scraped are coated with mineral oil. The site selected for scraping should be at the periphery of a lesion or the predilection site of the suspected parasite. The blade should be scraped back and forth over the skin until

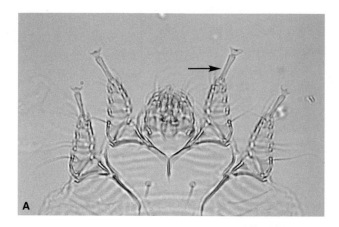

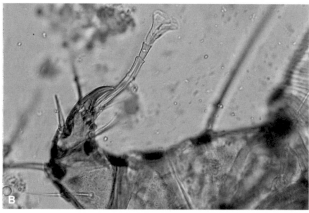

Fig. 4.1A and B. An important characteristic for identification of a number of common mites is length and segmentation of the stalk (pedicle) connecting a sucker to the leg. In *Sarcoptes* spp. mites (*A*), the stalk is long and unjointed (*arrow*). *Psoroptes* has a long, jointed pedicle (*B*).

Table 4.1. Microscopic characteristics of some mange, itch, and scab mites

	Leg Characteristics		
Genus	Egg-laying female	Male	Anus
Sarcoptes	Suckers on long, unsegmented stalks on pairs 1, 2; pointed scales on dorsum	Suckers on long unsegmented stalks on pairs 1, 2, 4; few pointed scales on dorsum	Terminal
Notoedres	Suckers as above; many prominent rounded scales on dorsum	Suckers as above; few rounded scales on dorsum	Dorsal
Knemidokoptes	No suckers	Suckers on unsegmented stalks on pairs 1, 2, 3, 4	Terminal
Psoroptes	Suckers on long, segmented stalks on pairs 1, 2, 4	Suckers on long, segmented stalks on pairs 1, 2, 3	Terminal
Chorioptes	Suckers on short, unsegmented stalks on pairs 1, 2, 4	Suckers on short, unsegmented stalks on pairs 1, 2, 3, 4; pair 4 rudimentary	Terminal
Otodectes	Suckers on short, unsegmented stalks on pairs 1, 2; pair 4 rudimentary	Suckers on short, unsegmented stalks on pairs 1, 2, 3, 4	Terminal
Trixacarus	Suckers on long, unsegmented stalks on pairs 1, 2		Dorsal

capillary bleeding is evident (a shallower scraping is done for surface-dwelling mites). For collection of *Demodex,* the follicle mite, a skin fold should be squeezed between the fingers to express the mites before the scraping is done. The debris collected on the scalpel blade is then placed on a microscope slide, coverslipped, and examined using the 10× microscope objective. Several slides may need to be examined before mites are found, especially in cases of *Sarcoptes* infestation.

To recover surface mites, such as *Cheyletiella,* a superficial scraping that does not cause bleeding is made with a scalpel blade coated in mineral oil. Alternatively, clear acetate tape can be used to collect material. The sticky side of the tape is pressed to the hair coat in an affected area and then placed on a microscope slide, trapping skin debris and mites against the slide and allowing microscopic examination. Brushings from the hair coat may also be examined.

If mites must be shipped to an acarologist or veterinary laboratory for identification, they should be stored in 70% alcohol. Skin scrapings and mites that are stored dry cannot usually be successfully identified.

PARASITE: *Sarcoptes scabiei* (Figures 4.2–4.5)

Common name: Itch mite (often called scabies mite in dogs).

Taxonomy: Mite (family Sarcoptidae).

Host: Host-specific varieties of *Sarcoptes* are found on a wide range of domestic animals, including dogs, ruminants, horses, rodents, swine, and camelids. Humans also have their own strain of *Sarcoptes.*

Geographic Distribution: Worldwide.

Location on Host: Hairless or thin-skinned areas of the body are usually the first to be affected, but large portions of the skin can be involved in severe cases.

Life Cycle: Transmission of *Sarcoptes* is by direct contact with an infested animal or fomites. Female mites tunnel into the epidermis, where eggs are deposited and where development of mites occurs. The life cycle from egg to adult occurs in about 3 weeks.

Laboratory Diagnosis: Deep skin scrapings are used for diagnosis. However, mites may be difficult to recover, and several scrapings should be collected from suspected cases. Many cases are treated presumptively when no mites are recovered. Fecal examination may reveal mites and mite eggs swallowed during grooming. In swine, *Sarcoptes* can often be found in scabs in the ears of chronically infected animals. To diagnose these infections on the farm, scab material can be removed and broken up over dark paper. Tiny, moving specks will be mites. Scabs can also be digested with 10% sodium hydroxide and the remaining material examined with the microscope. Characteristics of the terminal suckers used in identification are found in Table 4.1.

Size: Females approx. 400 µm, males approx. 250 µm

Clinical Importance: Mange caused by *Sarcoptes* is a highly pruritic condition accompanied by alopecia, thickening of the skin, and crust formation. In North America, infestations are most often encountered in dogs and swine, while other domestic animals are only rarely infested. *Sarcoptes* mites from animals can transiently infest humans and produce lesions.

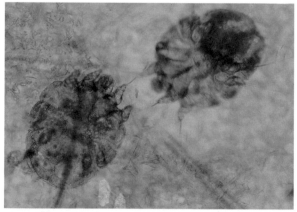

Fig. 4.2. *Sarcoptes* and related mites are typically round bodied. The third and fourth pairs of legs are short and often do not project beyond the margin of the body. Female *Sarcoptes* are approximately 400 µm in length; males are only about 250 µm long.

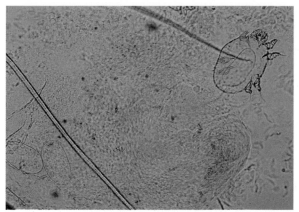

Fig. 4.3. Pruritic mite infestations may stimulate intense grooming by the host, resulting in the presence of both mites and their eggs in the feces. An egg is present in this female sarcoptic mite. These eggs are much larger than common helminth eggs (about 200 μm).

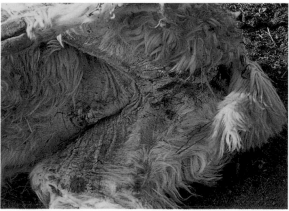

Fig. 4.4. *Sarcoptes scabiei* is a common cause of the condition called "scabies" in dogs. Lesions on the face and along the margin of the ear are common early in infestation. Photo courtesy of Dr. Jeffrey F. Williams, Vanson HaloSource, Inc., Redmond, WA.

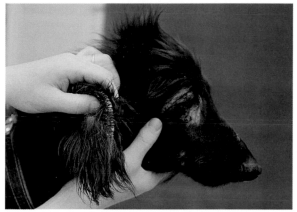

Fig. 4.5. Sarcoptic mange in an alpaca. In chronic sarcoptic mange, affected skin is hairless, thickened, and wrinkled. These nonspecific changes also occur in other chronic skin diseases. Photo courtesy of Dr. Jeffrey F. Williams, Vanson HaloSource, Inc., Redmond, WA.

PARASITE: *Notoedres* **spp.** (Figure 4.6)
        Common name: Ear mange mite (rodents).

Taxonomy: Mite (family Sarcoptidae).

Host: *Notoedres cati* occurs on cats. Other species occur on rodents, rabbits, and some wild animals.

Geographic Distribution: Worldwide.

Location on Host: The head is usually infested first, but mites may spread to other regions of the body.

Life Cycle: Similar to *Sarcoptes.*

Laboratory Diagnosis: Mites are observed with deep skin scrapings.

    Size: *N. cati* approx. 225 µm; rodent species are larger

Clinical Importance: Feline notoedric mange is usually confined to the head and neck. Infestations are rarely seen in North America.

PARASITE: *Knemidokoptes* **spp.** (Figures 4.7–4.8)
        Common name: Scaly leg or scaly face mite.

Taxonomy: Mite (family Knemidokoptidae).

Host: Birds, including domestic poultry and pet birds.

Geographic Distribution: Worldwide.

Location on Host: Nonfeathered portions of the body, including feet, legs, and face.

Life Cycle: Like *Sarcoptes,* transmission occurs by direct contact with infested birds or fomites, and all stages of the mite are found on the host.

Laboratory Diagnosis: Mites can be found in skin scrapings collected from the periphery of lesions. Typically, the exudative lesions produced by the mites contain numerous small holes, giving them a honeycombed appearance.

    Size: approx. 400 µm

Clinical Importance: *Knemidokoptes* species burrow under the scales on the legs or nonfeathered portions of the face, inducing a serous exudate that hardens into crusts. These proliferative lesions eventually may cause trauma and disfigurement leading to the death of the host.

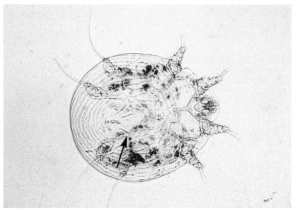

Fig. 4.6. *Notoedres* mites are similar in appearance to *Sarcoptes*. However, the anus of *Notoedres,* unlike that of *Sarcoptes,* is located on the dorsal surface (*arrow*) rather than the ventral. *Notoedres* also has scalloped scales on the dorsum rather than the sawtooth scales on *Sarcoptes*. The suckers on the front legs of *Notoedres* and *Sarcoptes* are attached to the legs by long, unjointed stalks.

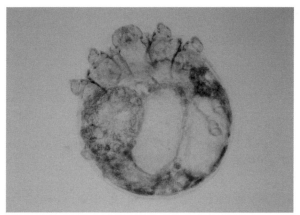

Fig. 4.7. *Knemidokoptes* is a round-bodied mite, generally similar in appearance to sarcoptic mites.

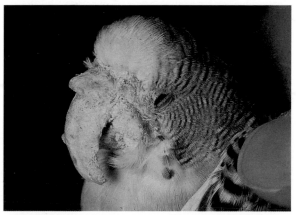

Fig. 4.8. Budgerigar with a deformed beak resulting from the proliferative lesion produced by *Knemidokoptes* infestation. Photo courtesy of Dr. Jeffrey F. Williams, Vanson HaloSource, Inc., Redmond WA.

PARASITE: *Trixacarus* **spp.** (Figure 4.9)

Taxonomy: Mite (family Sarcoptidae).

Host: Guinea pigs (*Trixacarus caviae*) and rats (*T. diversus*).

Geographic Distribution: Europe and North America.

Location on Host: Lesions begin on the head, neck, and back but can spread to other areas.

Life Cycle: Similar to *Sarcoptes*. Mites are readily transferred from the dam to young animals in the neonatal period.

Laboratory Diagnosis: Mites are identified in skin scrapings.

   Size: approx. 200 μm

Clinical Importance: *Trixacarus* is the sarcoptic mange mite of guinea pigs. Infestation is associated with pruritus, alopecia, and hyperkeratosis and can become a serious problem in guinea pig colonies. Humans in contact with infested guinea pigs may develop transient lesions.

PARASITE: *Psoroptes* **spp.** (Figures 4.10–4.13)
   Common name: Scab or scabies mite (ruminants).

Taxonomy: Mite (family Psoroptidae).

Host: *Psoroptes ovis* is the cause of psoroptic mange in ruminants; *P. cuniculi* (now thought to be a strain of *P. ovis*) is found on rabbits and ruminants. *Psoroptes* spp. can also be found on horses and some wildlife hosts. The number of species within the genus is currently undergoing revision.

Geographic Distribution: Worldwide.

Location on Host: *P. cuniculi* is found in the ears of rabbits, sheep, goats, and horses. Other *Psoroptes* infestations are often first detected on the dorsum of the host but may spread to other areas.

Life Cycle: Transmission is by direct contact or fomites. Unlike sarcoptic mites, *Psoroptes* spp. do not burrow, and all stages are found on the skin surface. The life cycle can be completed in as little as 10 days. Mites may survive for several days off the host.

Laboratory Diagnosis: Superficial skin scrapings should be collected from the periphery of skin lesions. Alternatively, skin scabs can be broken apart or digested and the residue examined microscopically. Crusts from the ears can be treated similarly when infestations of *P. cuniculi* are suspected. Psoroptic mites are more oval in shape and have longer legs than sarcoptic mites.

   Size: approx. 750 μm

Clinical Importance: *Psoroptes* is a highly contagious, economically important cause of skin disease in ruminants worldwide. Infestation leads to exudative dermatitis and hair loss. In the USA the strain of *P. ovis* affecting sheep has been eradicated, and the bovine strain has diminished in importance since the introduction of macrolide endectocide drugs. In severe cases, *P. cuniculi* lesions on rabbits may extend beyond the ears to the face, neck, and back.

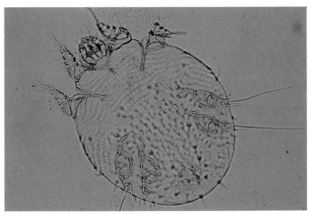

Fig. 4.9. Like other sarcoptic mites, *Trixacarus* is a round-bodied mite with short legs. *Trixacarus caviae* causes sarcoptic mange in guinea pigs.

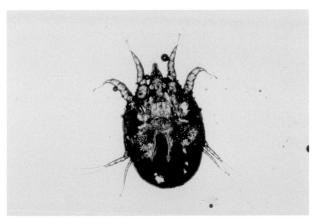

Fig. 4.10. Psoroptic mites have a more oval shape and longer legs than sarcoptic mites. Terminal suckers are connected to the legs by long, segmented stalks (Table 4.1). Photo courtesy of Dr. Robert Ridley, College of Veterinary Medicine, Kansas State University, Manhattan, KS.

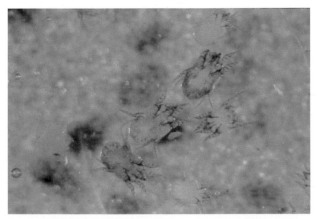

Fig. 4.11. *Psoroptes* may be up to 800 μm in length. Shown here are specimens of *Psoroptes cuniculi* from rabbit ears. Fig. 4.1B shows a closer view of the jointed pedicle on some of the legs of *Psoroptes*. Photo courtesy of Dr. David Baker, School of Veterinary Medicine, Louisiana State University, Baton Rouge, LA.

PARASITE: *Chorioptes bovis* (Figures 4.14–4.15)
> Common name: Foot mange, leg mange, itchy heel.

Taxonomy: Mite (family Psoroptidae).

Host: Varieties of *C. bovis* are found on ruminants, horses, and rabbits.

Geographic Distribution: Worldwide.

Location on Host: *Chorioptes* are found primarily on the lower body of the host. In horses, the mites are seen more often in breeds with feathered legs. In cattle, the rear legs, base of the tail, and back of the udder are most often affected.

Life Cycle: Transmission is by direct contact or fomites. *Chorioptes* mites spend their entire life cycle on the skin surface. The life cycle can be completed in about 3 weeks.

Laboratory Diagnosis: Mites are observed on skin scrapings. *Chorioptes* has short, unsegmented stalks bearing the suckers on the legs (see Table 4.1).

> Size: approx. 300 µm

Clinical Importance: Infestation may be asymptomatic or cause only mild lesions in some animals. As mite populations increase, pruritus, alopecia, and crusting may develop.

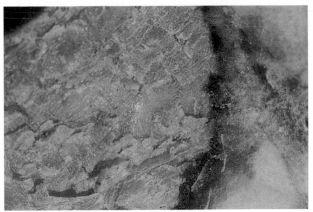

Fig. 4.12. Psorpotic mange or "scab" can be a serious infestation in ruminants. In sheep, mite activity causes an exudate that forms a crust on the surface of the skin, with the resulting loss of the fleece over affected areas. Photo courtesy of Dr. Jeffrey F. Williams, Vanson HaloSource, Inc., Redmond, WA.

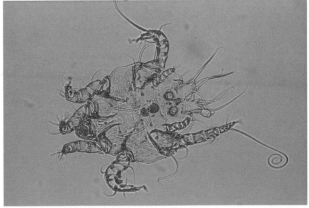

Fig. 4.13. Psoroptic ear mange in a rabbit. Photo courtesy of Dr. Jeffrey F. Williams, Vanson HaloSource, Inc., Redmond, WA.

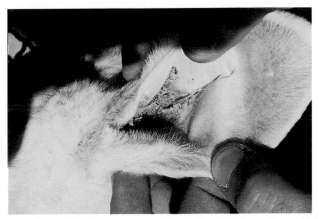

Fig. 4.14. *Chorioptes* is about 300 μm long. The two "eyes" on the posterior end of this *Chorioptes* male are actually copulatory suckers. Photo courtesy of Dr. Jeffrey F. Williams, Vanson HaloSource, Inc., Redmond, WA.

PARASITE: *Otodectes cynotis* (Figures 4.16–4.17)
           Common name: Ear mite.

Taxonomy: Mite (family Psoroptidae).

Host: Dogs, cats, and ferrets.

Geographic Distribution: Worldwide.

Location on Host: Ear canal.

Life Cycle: Mites complete their life cycle in the ear. Transmission occurs by direct contact or fomites. Kittens and puppies are easily infested by contact with the dam.

Laboratory Diagnosis: Routinely diagnosed by otoscope or microscopic examination of aural exudate collected with cotton swabs.

   Size: approx. 300 μm

Clinical Importance: These mites are a common cause of otitis externa. Bacterial decomposition of otic secretions and exudate leads to the formation of black, waxy cerumen. Infested animals often suffer severe pruritus that may lead to self-inflicted trauma. Heavy infestations may spread outside the ear to face, neck, and back.

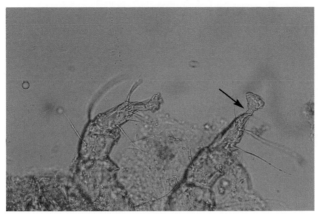

Fig. 4.15. *Chorioptes* mites are very similar in appearance to *Psoroptes* spp. The two genera can be accurately differentiated by the length and segmentation of the stalks (pedicles) carrying the suckers on the legs (Table 4.1). The suckers of *Chorioptes* are found on short, unsegmented stalks (*arrow*). See Fig. 4.1B for the pedicle of *Psoroptes.*

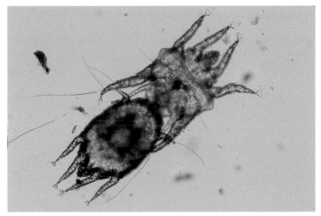

Fig. 4.16. Mating *Otodectes cynotis* mites from a ferret. *Otodectes* is another psoroptic mite with an oval-shaped body and long legs. They are similar in size and appearance to *Chorioptes*. In heavy infestations it is common to find copulating mites in ear swab preparations. The short unsegmented stalks carrying the suckers can be seen in this photo.

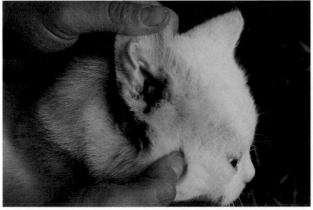

Fig. 4.17. *Otodectes cynotis* infestation in a cat. The mites cause the production of black "coffee ground" exudate. Photo courtesy of Dr. Jeffrey F. Williams, Vanson HaloSource, Inc., Redmond, WA.

Parasite: *Demodex* **spp.** (Figures 4.18–4.22)
        Common name: Follicle mite.

Taxonomy: Mite (family Demodicidae).

Host: Species of *Demodex* have been identified from many hosts, including dogs, cats, pigs, horses, cattle, goats, sheep, laboratory animals, humans, and other species.

Geographic Distribution: Worldwide.

Location on Host: Sebaceous glands and hair follicles.

Life Cycle: Mites are usually transferred from the dam to offspring in the neonatal period. All stages of the life cycle are found on the host.

Laboratory Diagnosis: Deep skin scrapings are required for diagnosis. A skin fold should be squeezed before scraping to express mites from follicles and sebaceous glands. Finding a high proportion of immature mites on a skin scraping is indicative of a more serious infestation than is a predominance of adult mites. *Demodex* and its eggs may be ingested during grooming by pruritic animals and be seen in fecal flotation tests.

    Size: 100–400 µm, depending on species

Clinical Importance: Most infested animals do not develop clinical disease. Dogs are the host most likely to be clinically affected. Generalized demodectic mange in dogs has a genetic component and is thought to be associated with an immune deficiency. Demodecosis is rare in livestock species.

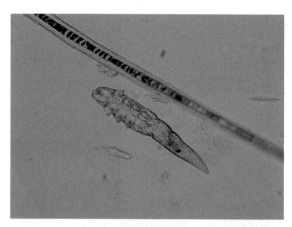

Fig. 4.18. *Demodex* spp. are usually described as looking like cigars with short legs. *Demodex canis*, shown in this photo, reaches a length of about 390 µm.

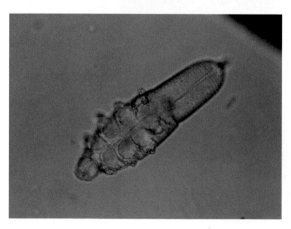

Fig. 4.19. Many animals are parasitized by *Demodex* spp. Shown here is *Demodex* from a gerbil. Hosts rarely show clinical signs of infestation. Photo courtesy of Dr. David Baker, School of Veterinary Medicine, Louisiana State University, Baton Rouge, LA.

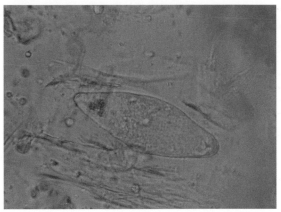

Fig. 4.20. *Demodex* egg in a canine skin scraping. Both mites and eggs may be detected in feces when pruritic animals swallow the parasites during grooming.

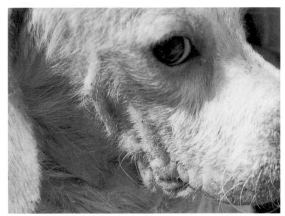

Fig. 4.21. *Demodex* is most often seen as a clinical problem in dogs. Lesions often appear first on the face or forelegs. Photo courtesy of Dr. Jeffrey F. Williams, Vanson HaloSource, Inc., Redmond, WA.

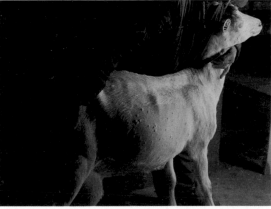

Fig. 4.22. In goats clinical demodecosis is usually associated with the formation of pustules. Photo courtesy of Dr. Jeffrey F. Williams, Vanson HaloSource, Inc., Redmond, WA, and Dr. C. S. F. Williams, Langley, WA.

PARASITE: *Cheyletiella* **spp.** (Figures 4.23–4.24)
Common name: Walking dandruff.

Taxonomy: Mite (family Cheyletiellidae).

Host: *Cheyletiella parasitovorax, C. yasguri,* and *C. blakei* are seen on rabbits, dogs, and cats respectively.

Geographic Distribution: Worldwide.

Location on Host: *Cheyletiella* infestations are usually seen on the back. In cats, the head is also often affected.

Life Cycle: Transmission is by direct contact or fomites. *Cheyletiella* can be carried from one animal to another by fleas (*Ctenocephalides*). Mites can live up to 10 days in the environment.

Laboratory Diagnosis: *Cheyletiella* is a fur mite and not a skin dweller, so only superficial skin scrapings are required for diagnosis. Alternatively, if material combed from the hair is examined against a dark background, mites can be seen as moving white dots ("walking dandruff"). The distinctive feature of the mite is the large palpal claws.

Size: approx. 400 μm

Clinical Importance: Many infested animals do not show clinical signs. Young animals are most likely to show evidence of infestation, including crusting, increased skin scurf, and pruritus. In heavy infestations hair loss may occur. Owners may develop lesions in areas of close contact with their animals.

PARASITE: *Lynxacarus radovskyi* (Figure 4.25)

Taxonomy: Mite (family Listrophoridae).

Host: Cats; other species infest bobcats and weasels.

Geographic Distribution: Australia, southern USA, Caribbean, and Hawaii.

Location on Host: Mites clasp the hairs of cats, primarily on the tail head, tail tip, and in the perineal area.

Life Cycle: The entire life cycle is spent on the host. Infestation is by direct contact.

Laboratory Diagnosis: Laterally flattened mites can be seen clinging to cat hairs. Eggs are attached to the hairs.

Size: approx. 450 μm

Clinical Importance: Heavy mite infestations can affect the entire body and lead to poor condition of the hair coat. This mite is rare in North America.

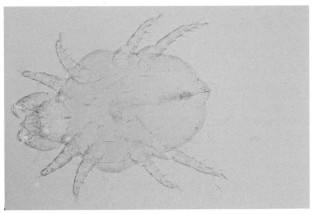

Fig. 4.23. *Cheyletiella* is a surface mite that can be collected by brushing the hair coat or collecting material with sticky tape. In heavy infestations mites may be found throughout the hair coat.

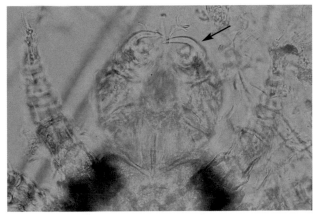

Fig. 4.24. *Cheyletiella* spp. are easily identified microscopically by the presence of large palpal claws (*arrow*). Small combs are found on the legs instead of the suckers seen in some other species of parasitic mites.

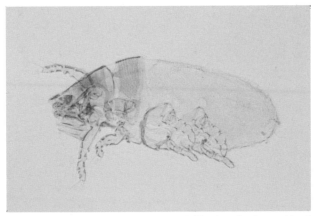

Fig. 4.25. The body of the *Lynxacarus* mite is laterally compressed, like that of a flea, and has large sternal plates that are used, along with the first two sets of legs, to encircle the hair.

PARASITE: *Leporacarus* (= *Listrophorus*) *gibbus* (Figures 4.26–4.27)
> Common name: Fur mite.

Taxonomy: Mite (family Listrophoridae). This mite formerly belonged to the genus *Listrophorus*.

Host: Rabbits.

Geographic Distribution: Worldwide.

Location on Host: Throughout the fur.

Life Cycle: Transmission is by direct contact. All stages of the life cycle are found on the host.

Laboratory Diagnosis: Mites are large enough to be seen as small specks on the hairs and can be collected by combing and examining hairs with a magnifying glass or microscope.

> Size: approx. 350–500 μm

Clinical Importance: Mites usually cause no clinical signs even though large numbers may be present.

PARASITE: *Chirodiscoides caviae* (Figure 4.28)
> Common name: Fur mite.

Taxonomy: Mite (family Listrophoridae).

Host: Guinea pigs.

Geographic Distribution: Worldwide.

Location on Host: Attached to hairs.

Life Cycle: Transmission is by direct contact with an infested individual or fomite.

Laboratory Diagnosis: Mites are detected by examining hairs from the host.

> Size: approx. 500 μm

Clinical Importance: This mite is considered generally nonpathogenic.

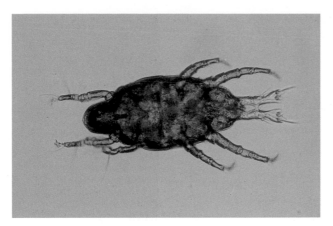

Fig. 4.26. Male *Leporacarus* (10×) mites are laterally compressed and have a brown anterior shield that contrasts with the white idiosoma. The palps are modified to form two chitinous flaps used for attachment to hairs.

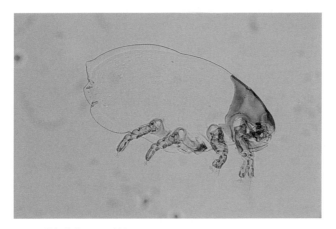

Fig. 4.27. Female *Leporacarus* (40×) from a rabbit.

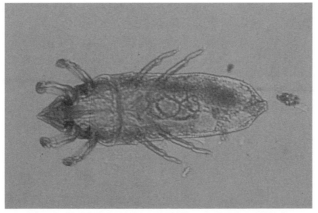

Fig. 4.28. *Chirodiscoides* from a guinea pig. The mite is about 500 μm in length, and the first two pairs of legs are adapted for wrapping around the hair shafts of the host. Photo courtesy of Dr. David Baker, School of Veterinary Medicine, Louisiana State University, Baton Rouge, LA.

PARASITE: *Mycoptes musculinus, Myobia musculi, Radfordia* **spp.** (Figures 4.29–4.30)
Common name: Fur mite.

Taxonomy: Mites (families Listrophoridae and Myobidae).

Host: Mice and rats.

Geographic Distribution: Worldwide.

Location on Host: Hair coat.

Life Cycle: Transmission is by direct contact; all stages of the life cycle are found on the host.

Laboratory Diagnosis: Diagnosis is made by detecting mites on host hairs.

Size:	*Radfordia* and *Myobia*	approx. 400–450 μm
	Mycoptes	approx. 350 μm

Clinical Importance: Some infested animals tolerate large numbers of mites without clinical signs, although pruritus, erythema, hair loss, and thickened skin may occur in others. Secondary bacterial infections may develop.

PARASITE: Avian Feather Mites (Figure 4.31)

Taxonomy: Mites (numerous families and species).

Host: Domestic and wild birds.

Geographic Distribution: Worldwide.

Location on Host: Species specialized for different feather environments.

Life Cycle: Most mites live on the feather surface and feed on secretions and skin and feather debris. Quill mites live in the base of the feathers and feed on host tissue or fluids.

Laboratory Diagnosis: Diagnosis is made by detection and identification of mites on feathers.

Size: variable with species

Clinical Importance: Most feather mite infestations appear to cause little damage and are usually considered of minor clinical importance.

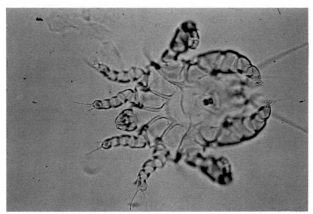

Fig. 4.29. *Mycoptes musculinus* from the hair coat of a mouse. In males the fourth pair of legs is enlarged and directed backward. Photo courtesy of Dr. David Baker, School of Veterinary Medicine, Louisiana State University, Baton Rouge, LA.

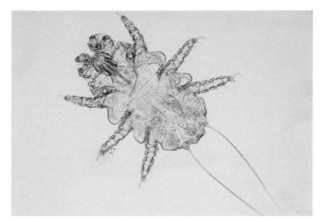

Fig. 4.30. *Radfordia* is found at the base of the hairs. The first pair of legs is modified for feeding and projects forward. *Radfordia* is similar in appearance to another rodent fur mite, *Myobia musculi*. However, *Radfordia* has two claws on the second pair of legs, while *Myobia* has only one claw.

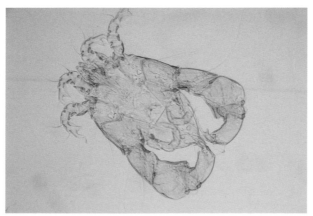

Fig. 4.31. Male *Mesalgoides* sp. mite from a wild bird. Feather mite species show great variation in morphology as a result of specialization for life in different parts of the avian feather environment.

PARASITE: *Ornithonyssus sylviarum, O. bursa* (Figures 4.32–4.33)
        Common name: Northern fowl mite, tropical fowl mite.

Taxonomy: Mite (order Mesostigmata).

Geographic Distribution: The northern fowl mite, *O. sylviarum,* is found in temperate regions worldwide. The tropical fowl mite, *O. bursa*, is found in tropical and subtropical climates. Both species are found in the USA.

Location on Host: Mites and egg masses can be found on the skin among the feathers. In poultry, *O. sylviarum* often concentrates around the vent, causing a dark discoloration of the area.

Life Cycle: *Ornithonyssus sylviarum* spends its life on the avian host, whereas individuals of *O. bursa* spend greater periods of time off the host. Wild birds can introduce the mites into poultry facilities. Under appropriate conditions, the life cycle of *O. sylviarum* can be completed in a week.

Laboratory Diagnosis: Large mites are observed on birds or in the environment.

    Size: approx. 750 μm

Clinical Importance: Scabbing and matted feathers can develop on infested birds. In severe cases anemia, decreased production, and death may occur. Mites can act as vectors of other avian disease agents, including those causing Newcastle disease and fowl pox. Humans in contact with mites may also develop lesions.

PARASITE: *Ornithonyssus bacoti* (Figures 4.32–4.33)
        Common name: Tropical rat mite.

Taxonomy: Mite (order Mesostigmata).

Host: Rodents, occasionally other animals and humans.

Geographic Distribution: Worldwide.

Location on Host: Skin.

Life Cycle: Adult mites lay eggs in the environment. Mites visit the host only to feed; they spend the rest of the time in the host's bedding or nest. The life cycle can be completed in about 2 weeks.

Laboratory Diagnosis: Mites on animals or in the environment are observed.

    Size: approx. 750 μm

Clinical Importance: In large numbers, this blood-feeding mite can cause anemia, debilitation, and even death. Humans in contact with infested laboratory or pet rodents may develop lesions.

PARASITE: *Dermanyssus gallinae* (Figure 4.34)
        Common name: Red poultry mite.

Taxonomy: Mite (order Mesostigmata).

Host: Wild and domestic birds.

Geographic Distribution: Worldwide.

Location on Host: Mites can occur anywhere on the body.

Life Cycle: Mites visit the host at night only to take blood meals. During the day, the mites are found in crevices in the environment. The life cycle can be completed in as little as 10 days. Adults can survive in the environment for several months without feeding.

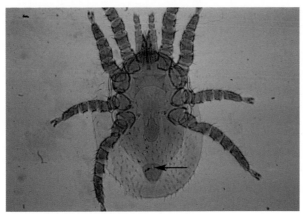

Fig. 4.32. *Ornithonyssus* spp. belong to the mesostigmatid order of mites. These mites have long legs in the anterior portion of the body and are more ticklike in appearance than other mites. In *Ornithonyssus* spp., the anus (*arrow*) is at the anterior end of the anal plate. The anus of *Dermanyssus gallinae*, a morphologically similar mite, is located in the posterior portion of the anal plate. Photo courtesy of Dr. David Baker, School of Veterinary Medicine, Louisiana State University, Baton Rouge, LA.

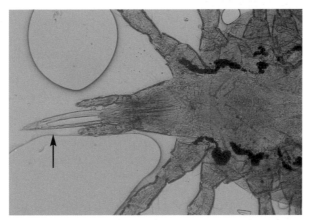

Fig. 4.33. Another characteristic used to differentiate *Ornithonyssus* from the similar genus *Dermanyssus* is the chelicerae (*arrow*). The chelicerae in this *Ornithonyssus* mite are shorter than the long, whiplike chelicerae of *Dermanyssus.*

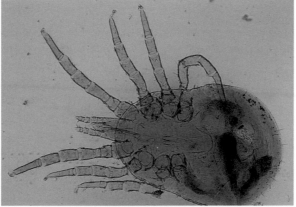

Fig. 4.34. *Dermanyssus gallinae* infests both domestic and wild birds. The anus of this mite is present in a more posterior position on the anal plate than in *Ornithonyssus*. *Dermanyssus gallinae* also has long, whiplike chelicerae (not visible in this figure). Differentiating the genera may be helpful in determining appropriate control measures because of differences in life cycles.

Laboratory Diagnosis: Mite infestation may be difficult to diagnose because the mites are not on the host during the day. Close examination of the environment may reveal mites under crusts of manure on perches or in nest boxes. If infestation is suspected in caged birds, the cage can be covered with a white cloth at night. In the morning mites will be seen as small black or dark red dots clinging to the cloth.

Size: approx. 750 μm

Clinical Importance: Heavy infestation can cause anemia and death, particularly in hatchlings. Hens may be reluctant to sit on their nests. Other animals and humans in close proximity to infested birds or their nests may also be attacked and develop lesions.

PARASITE: *Pneumonyssoides caninum* (Figure 4.35)
　　　　Common name: Nasal mite.

Taxonomy: Mite (order Mesostigmata).

Host: Dogs. A similar mite, *Pneumonyssus simicola,* parasitizes the respiratory system of some monkey species.

Geographic Distribution: Worldwide.

Location on Host: Nasal sinuses of dogs.

Life Cycle: The life cycle of this mite is poorly understood, but transmission is thought to be by direct contact since mites are sometimes seen crawling on the nose.

Laboratory Diagnosis: Mites are observed in the nasal sinuses and passages or crawling outside the nostrils.

Size: approx. 1 mm

Clinical Importance: Infestations are usually asymptomatic but may produce sneezing, rhinitis, sinusitis, and malaise. In captive monkeys, *Pneumonyssus* can cause significant respiratory disease.

PARASITE: **Trombiculid Mites** (Figures 4.36–4.37)
　　　　Common name: Chigger, harvest mite, scrub itch mite.

Taxonomy: Mites (family Trombiculidae).

Host: Wide variety of animals and humans.

Geographic Distribution: Several species parasitize a variety of hosts, including *Eutrombicula alfreddugesi, E. splendens* (North America), and *Neotrombicula autumnalis* (Europe).

Location on Host: Predilection sites include the face, head, and legs.

Life Cycle: Only the larval stage of chigger mites is parasitic. Eggs are laid in the environment. Larvae attach to a host and feed for 3–5 days and then complete development in the environment. Adults are predators of other arthropods.

Laboratory Diagnosis: Small, often orange or red mites are often seen in clusters on the face of the host. The presence of only larval stages is helpful in diagnosing chigger infestations.

Size: approx. 200–500 μm, depending on species

Clinical Importance: Mites may cause pruritus and irritation. Humans are also susceptible to infestation, with pruritic lesions frequently appearing in areas where clothing is constrictive (i.e., at the waistband of pants, top of socks, etc.).

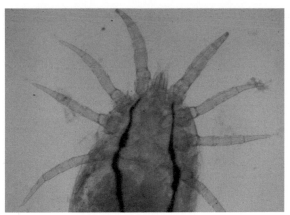

Fig. 4.35. *Pneumonyssoides caninum*, the nasal mite of dogs. A related mite, *Pneumonyssus simicola*, is the lung mite of several species of African monkeys. Photo courtesy of Dr. Jeffrey F. Williams, Vanson HaloSource, Inc., Redmond, WA.

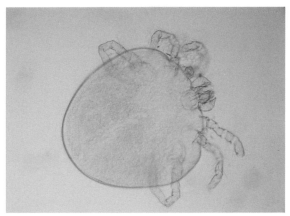

Fig. 4.36. Only the six-legged larvae of chiggers are parasitic, which is helpful in identification of the parasites. This *Blankaartia* sp chigger was removed from a bird.

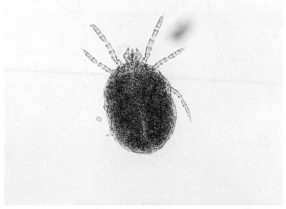

Fig. 4.37. Specimen of *Trombicula* sp., a cause of mammalian chigger infestation. Photo courtesy of Dr. Jeffrey F. Williams, Vanson HaloSource, Inc., Redmond, WA.

Tick Identification

Ticks are usually larger than mites, ranging in length from 3 to 12 mm, or more in the case of engorged females. Ticks are divided into two families: Ixodidae (hard ticks) and Argasidae (soft ticks). The Ixodid (hard) ticks are of greatest importance in veterinary medicine. Various hard tick species are vectors of a number of viral, bacterial, and protozoal animal and human pathogens. In addition, hard tick species cause tick paralysis and tick toxicosis.

All ticks pass from the egg through larval and nymphal stages before becoming adults and utilize one or more host animals during the developmental cycle. Eggs are always laid in the environment. Hard tick larvae are acquired by the host from the environment. All hard ticks undergo a single molt from the larval to the nymphal stage and a second molt from the nymph to the adult. These molts follow attachment and blood feeding on the host that usually lasts for several days. Tick species that remain on the host during the two molting periods are known as one-host ticks. In two-host tick species, the molt to the nymphal stage occurs on the host, but the engorged nymph leaves the host, molts in the environment and then finds a new host. In the three-host tick life cycle, both the larva and nymph leave the host to molt, attaching to a host again after each molt. In some cases, each tick stage prefers the same host species; in others, host preference may vary with the stage of the tick. In much of North America, the most important tick species are three-host ticks. Soft tick life cycles are more variable than those of the hard ticks. Many soft tick species live in the environment and visit the host only briefly to take repeated blood meals.

All stages of ticks are large enough to be grossly visible on animals, although larvae may be only a few millimeters in length and soft ticks usually do not attach for long periods. Hard ticks are likely to be found attached in areas on the host that cannot be easily groomed, for example, the head, neck, and ears of most host species, and also the tail of horses (Fig. 4.38). Because ticks are important vectors of zoonotic diseases (Lyme disease, Rocky Mountain spotted fever, etc.), they should be removed using forceps or tweezers instead of the fingers to reduce the possibility of contact with tick body fluids containing infectious organisms. The tick should be firmly grasped directly behind the point of attachment to the skin and then pulled off. Often a small portion of skin will also be pulled away.

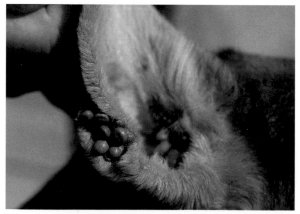

Fig. 4.38. Ticks are most often found attached on parts of the body that are difficult for the host to groom. Unidentified ticks are attached to the ear of this dog. Photo courtesy of Dr. Jeffrey F. Williams, Vanson HaloSource, Inc., Redmond, WA.

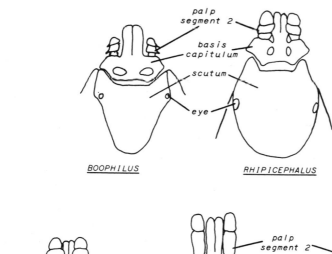

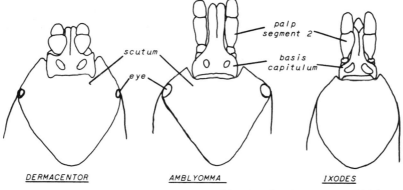

Fig. 4.39. Comparison of the basis capitulum and mouthparts of females of the important Ixodid tick genera of domestic animals in North America. The scutum of the adult male hard ticks covers the entire dorsum of the parasite.

Hard ticks have a hard dorsal shield called the scutum. The scutum is limited to the anterior, central region of the dorsum in females, whereas in males the scutum extends over the entire dorsal region. The mouthparts of hard ticks are evident from the dorsal surface. The Argasid (soft) ticks have a leathery integument, which often is spinose or bumpy. The mouthparts of soft ticks can be seen only from the ventral aspect of the tick.

Identification of adult hard ticks to the level of genus is not difficult in a veterinary practice. One of the most useful characteristics for identifying the genus of a hard tick is the shape of the basis capitulum and mouthparts. Figure 4.39 shows these characteristics on adult females; a magnifying glass is useful for looking at the basis capitulum. The pigmented markings of the scutum (referred to as "ornamentation") are another useful characteristic. Ticks with ornamentation are called "ornate"; those lacking these markings are "inornate." Additionally, in some genera, the posterior margin of the body has a series of indentations, known as festoons. Features like festoons are much more difficult to appreciate on engorged female ticks. Identification is easiest with unengorged females or males. Nymphs, like adults, have eight legs but lack the genital pore seen in adults. Using these characteristics, a dichotomous key for the genera of adult ticks (Fig. 4.40) can be followed for identification of most tick specimens in North America. Identification of six-legged larval ticks is more difficult and may require the assistance of an expert.

If specific identification of ticks is required, they should be preserved and submitted in 70–80% alcohol.

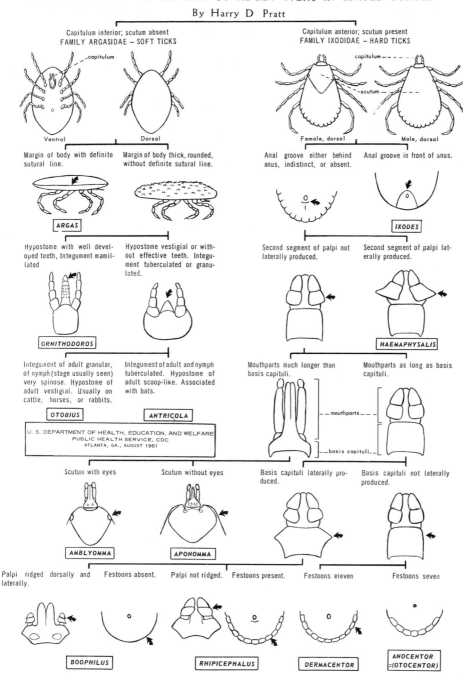

PICTORIAL KEY TO GENERA OF ADULT TICKS IN UNITED STATES
By Harry D Pratt

Capitulum inferior; scutum absent
FAMILY ARGASIDAE – SOFT TICKS

Capitulum anterior; scutum present
FAMILY IXODIDAE – HARD TICKS

capitulum

scutum

Ventral   Dorsal   Female, dorsal   Male, dorsal

Margin of body with definite sutural line.

Margin of body thick, rounded, without definite sutural line.

Anal groove either behind anus, indistinct, or absent.

Anal groove in front of anus.

ARGAS   **IXODES**

Hypostome with well developed teeth, Integument mamillated

Hypostome vestigial or without effective teeth. Integument tuberculated or granulated.

Second segment of palpi not laterally produced.

Second segment of palpi laterally produced.

ORNITHODOROS   **HAEMAPHYSALIS**

Integument of adult granular, of nymph (stage usually seen) very spinose. Hypostome of adult vestigial. Usually on cattle, horses, or rabbits.

Integument of adult and nymph tuberculated. Hypostome of adult scoop-like. Associated with bats.

Mouthparts much longer than basis capituli.

Mouthparts as long as basis capituli.

OTOBIUS   **ANTRICOLA**

U. S. DEPARTMENT OF HEALTH, EDUCATION, AND WELFARE
PUBLIC HEALTH SERVICE, CDC
ATLANTA, GA., AUGUST 1961

— mouthparts — —

— basis capituli —

Scutum with eyes   Scutum without eyes

Basis capituli laterally produced.

Basis capituli not laterally produced.

AMBLYOMMA   **APONOMMA**

Palpi ridged dorsally and laterally.

Festoons absent.   Palpi not ridged.   Festoons present.   Festoons eleven   Festoons seven

BOOPHILUS   **RHIPICEPHALUS**   **DERMACENTOR**   **ANOCENTOR =(OTOCENTOR)**

X - 30

Fig. 4.40. Key to adult tick genera found in North America. Examination of ticks with low magnification should allow identification of features used in this key. Courtesy of US Public Health Service, CDC.

PARASITE: *Amblyomma* spp. (Figures 4.41–4.44)
        Common name: Lone Star tick, Gulf Coast tick, bont tick.

Taxonomy: Tick (family Ixodidae).

Host: A wide variety of domestic and wild animals serve as hosts.

Geographic Distribution: Approximately 100 species are found predominantly in tropical and sub-tropical areas. Tropical species important in domestic animals include *A. hebraeum* (bont tick) and *A. variegatum* (tropical bont tick). *Amblyomma americanum* (Lone Star tick) and *A. maculatum* (Gulf Coast tick) are common species in the USA.

Location on Host: Various, often found on domestic animals in the head and neck region.

Life Cycle: *Amblyomma* spp. are three-host ticks, meaning that each stage of the life cycle must find a new host following a molt in the environment. Larvae and nymphs feed on a wide variety of hosts; adults are often found on ruminants and other domestic animals and humans.

Laboratory Diagnosis: Long mouthparts are an important diagnostic feature of *Amblyomma*. The scutum is usually ornamented.

Clinical Importance: The long mouthparts of *Amblyomma* make attachment particularly painful and susceptible to secondary infection. Economic loss from damaged hides may occur. *Amblyomma americanum* is a vector of the bacteria causing tularemia and Q fever and several *Ehrlichia* species. In Africa, *A. hebraeum* and *A. variegatum* transmit heartwater (*Cowdria*), tick-bite fever (*Rickettsia conori*), and Nairobi sheep disease (Nairovirus). *Amblyomma variegatum* also transmits heartwater in the Caribbean.

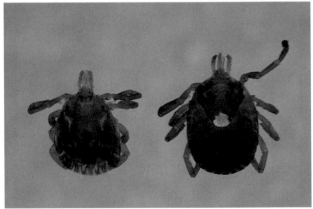

Fig. 4.41. Male and female *Amblyomma americanum* (Lone Star tick). The female (*right*) of this common US tick is easily recognized by the presence of the large white spot at the posterior margin of the scutum. Males do not have any conspicuous markings on the scutum.

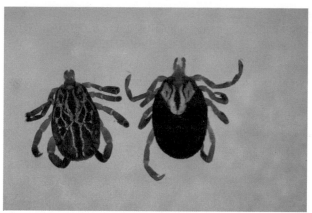

Fig. 4.42. *Amblyomma maculatum:* (*left*) male; (*right*) female. The Gulf Coast tick is found in the southeastern USA and Mexico. It feeds primarily on the head and neck of birds and mammals. Note the long mouthparts typical of this genus.

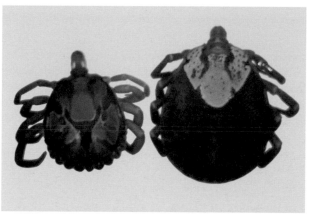

Fig. 4.43. *Amblyomma* spp. are common in the tropics and subtropics. They are often highly ornamented with iridescent markings like these African *Amblyomma*. Some tick genera, like *Amblyomma*, have simple eyes on the margin of the scutum (see Fig. 4.39).

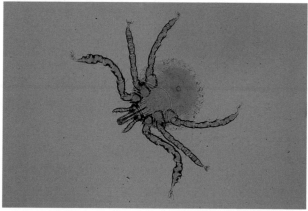

Fig. 4.44. Larval or seed tick, so called because of their small size. This tick has been treated with a clearing solution. Larval ticks are much smaller than adults and have only six legs. Seed ticks of some species may attach in large numbers to domestic animals or humans.

PARASITE: *Ixodes* spp. (Figures 4.45–4.47, 4.55)

    Common name: Black-legged tick, deer tick, European sheep tick (castor bean tick), hedgehog tick, British dog tick, Australian and South African paralysis ticks.

Taxonomy: Tick (family Ixodidae). *Ixodes* is the largest genus of hard ticks, containing more than 200 species.

Host: Many host species, including domestic animals and humans.

Geographic Distribution: Some of the most important species in domestic animals include *I. scapularis* (black-legged or deer tick) and *I. pacificus* (western black-legged tick) in North America; *I. ricinus* (sheep or castor bean tick), *I. canisuga* (British dog tick), and *I. hexagonus* (hedgehog tick) in Europe; *I. rubicundus* (South African paralysis tick) and *I. holocyclus* (Australian paralysis tick).

Location on Host: Various.

Life Cycle: *Ixodes* species are three-host ticks.

Laboratory Diagnosis: The most helpful characteristic for identification of *Ixodes* ticks is an anal groove that runs from the posterior margin of the body to just anterior to the anus. A magnifying glass or dissecting type microscope may be needed to appreciate this feature.

Clinical Importance: *Ixodes* spp. in North America and Europe are vectors of Lyme borreliosis and several species of *Ehrlichia*. *Ixodes ricinus* also transmits louping-ill and *Babesia* spp. in Europe. Species of this genus can also cause dermatitis and tick worry and are major causes of tick paralysis in Australia and South Africa.

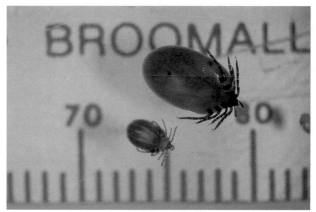

Fig. 4.45. Nymph and adult female *Ixodes scapularis,* the deer tick. This species is the primary vector of Lyme disease in the USA and is smaller than other common ticks.

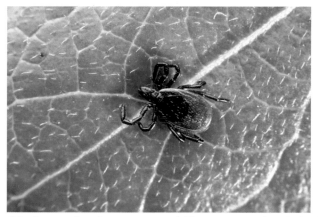

Fig. 4.46. The scutum of *Ixodes scapularis* is not ornamented. Photo courtesy of Agricultural Research Service, US Department of Agriculture.

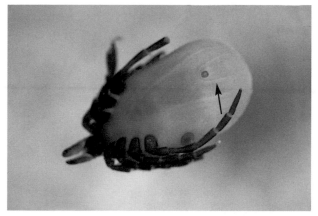

Fig. 4.47. The distinctive morphologic detail of the *Ixodes* ticks is the groove that runs anterior to the anus (*arrow*). In other tick genera, this groove is posterior to the anus or absent. *Ixodes* ticks also have long mouthparts.

PARASITE: *Dermacentor* spp. (Figures 4.48–4.49)
>   Common name: American dog tick, Rocky Mountain wood tick, winter tick, tropical horse tick.

Taxonomy: Tick (family Ixodidae).

Host: Depending on the species, a wide variety of wild and domestic hosts can be used.

Geographic Distribution: Primarily Europe, Asia, and North America. *Dermacentor variabilis* (American dog tick), *D. andersoni* (Rocky Mountain wood tick), *D. albipictus* (winter or elk or horse tick), and *D. occidentalis* (Pacific Coast tick) are found in North America and parasitize a variety of animals. *Dermacentor nitens* is a parasite of equids in Florida, the Caribbean, and Latin America. In Europe, *D. reticulatus* is an important species.

Location on Host: Various.

Life Cycle: Most *Dermacentor* spp. are three-host ticks that prefer small rodents in larval and nymphal stages and larger vertebrates in the adult stage. *Dermacentor nitens and D. albipictus* are one-host ticks.

Laboratory Diagnosis: *Dermacentor* spp. are usually ornamented with relatively short mouthparts and a rectangular basis capitulum.

Clinical Importance: *Dermacentor* spp. in the USA are the most common vectors of Rocky Mountain spotted fever and can also transmit anaplasmosis to cattle. *Dermacentor nitens* is the vector of equine˙babesiosis in the USA. In Europe, *D. reticulatus* is the vector of equine and canine babesiosis. Several species of *Dermacentor* are known to cause tick paralysis.

PARASITE: *Rhipicephalus* spp. (Figures 4.50–4.51)
>   Common name: Brown dog tick or kennel tick, brown ear tick, red-legged tick.

Taxonomy: Tick (family Ixodidae). Important parasites of domestic animals include *R. sanguineus* (brown dog tick), *R. appendiculatus* (brown ear tick), and *R. evertsi* (red-legged tick).

Host: This genus is most important in cattle and dogs.

Geographic Distribution: *Rhipicephalus sanguineus* is found worldwide. *Rhipicephalus appendiculatus* and *R. evertsi* are found on livestock in Africa.

Location on Host: Various.

Life Cycle: *Rhipicephalus sanguineus* is a three-host tick that uses a dog host for each stage of the life cycle. *Rhipicephalus appendiculatus* is also a three-host tick, while *R. evertsi* is a two-host tick.

Laboratory Diagnosis: *Rhipicephalus* spp. have a hexagonally shaped basis capitulum.

Clinical Importance: *Rhipicephalus sanguineus* transmits *Babesia canis* and *Ehrlichia canis* to dogs. *Rhipicephalus appendiculatus* and *R. evertsi* are the primary vectors of bovine theileriosis and also transmit babesiosis and Nairobi sheep disease to livestock.

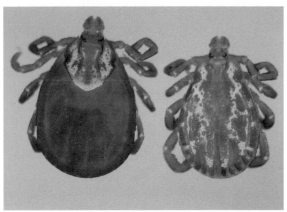

Fig. 4.48. *Dermacentor variabilis:* (*left*) female; (*right*) male. Like many members of this genus, *D. variabilis* (the American dog tick) is an ornamented tick. The short mouthparts, rectangular shape of the basis capitulum, and presence of festoons are used in identifying the genus.

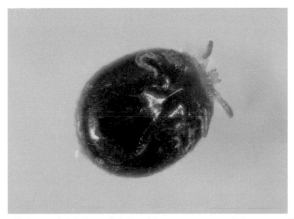

Fig. 4.49. Larval tick, also called a seed tick. Larval ticks of *Dermacentor variabilis* are usually found on wild rodents.

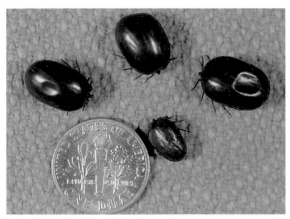

Fig. 4.50. Engorged female *Rhipicephalus sanguineus* (brown dog tick). This species is not ornamented. In the USA, it is most common in southern states but can also be a pest in kennels in other areas since dogs are used as hosts for every stage of the life cycle. Photo courtesy of Dr. Jeffrey F. Williams, Vanson HaloSource, Inc., Redmond, WA.

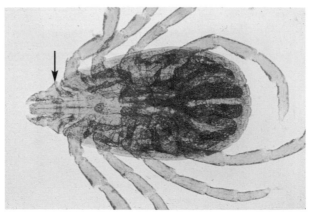

Fig. 4.51. The brown dog tick, *Rhipicephalus sanguineus.* Members of this tick genus have a basis capitulum that is hexagonal in shape with flared sides (*arrow;* see also Fig. 4.39). Photo courtesy of Dr. Byron Blagburn, College of Veterinary Medicine, Auburn University, Auburn, AL.

PARASITE: *Boophilus* spp. (Figures 4.52–4.53, 4.55)
        Common name: Cattle fever tick, blue tick, tropical cattle tick.

Taxonomy: Tick (family Ixodidae).

Host: This small genus contains several important parasites of cattle. Other animals may also serve as hosts.

Geographic Distribution: *Boophilus microplus* (tropical cattle tick) is found worldwide; *B. annulatus* (cattle fever tick) is found in the Western Hemisphere and parts of Africa; *B. decoloratus* (blue tick) is an African tick.

Location on Host: Various.

Life Cycle: *Boophilus* spp. are one-host ticks. After hatching from the egg in the environment, ticks locate a host, where they remain through the subsequent nymphal and adult stages. Females leave the host to lay their eggs in the environment.

Laboratory Diagnosis: *Boophilus* ticks can be identified by the presence of ridged palps and the absence of festoons.

Clinical Importance: *Boophilus* spp. are the intermediate hosts and vectors of bovine babesiosis. This important disease of cattle has been eradicated from the USA but remains prevalent in many other countries. *Boophilus* spp. also serve as vectors of bovine anaplasmosis.

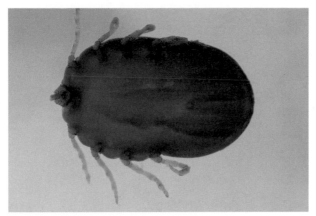

Fig. 4.52. Engorged female *Boophilus* sp. This genus lacks festoons and has distinctive ridged palps.

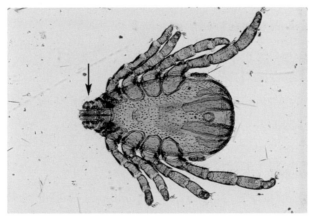

Fig. 4.53. The ridged palps of *Boophilus* (*arrow*) can be seen more clearly in this cleared specimen. Photo courtesy of Dr. Jeffrey F. Williams, Vanson HaloSource, Inc., Redmond, WA.

Parasite: *Haemaphysalis* **spp.** (Figures 4.54–4.55)
   Common name: Rabbit tick, yellow dog tick.

Taxonomy: Tick (family Ixodidae).

Host: *Haemaphysalis* ticks parasitize a wide range of mammals and birds, depending on species.

Geographic Distribution: Worldwide. *Haemaphysalis leporispalustris* (rabbit tick) is found in the Western Hemisphere, *H. punctata* is a parasite of livestock in Eurasia and North Africa, and *H. leachi* is the yellow dog tick found in Africa and parts of Asia.

Location on Host: Various.

Life Cycle: *Haemaphysalis* spp. are three-host ticks and leave the host after each blood meal.

Laboratory Diagnosis: Ticks of this genus have festoons, and the second segment of the palps flares out on the lateral margin.

Clinical Importance: Large numbers of *Haemaphysalis* ticks contribute to poor condition and "tick worry." *Haemaphysalis punctata* can transmit several species of *Babesia* and anaplasmosis to livestock. *Haemaphysalis leachi* is a vector of canine babesiosis. This genus is of minor importance in North America.

Parasite: *Argas* **spp.** (Figure 4.56)
   Common name: Fowl tick.

Taxonomy: Tick (family Argasidae). Important species include *A. persicus* and *A. reflexus.*

Host: Poultry and wild birds.

Geographic Distribution: Worldwide.

Location on Host: Various.

Life Cycle: *Argas* is a soft tick that lives in the environment, attacking birds only to feed, usually during the night. Several blood meals are taken by larval and adult ticks.

Laboratory Diagnosis: As their name suggests, soft ticks lack the hard "enameled" appearance of hard ticks. The mouthparts of soft ticks cannot be seen from the dorsal surface, which also helps to distinguish them from hard ticks. *Argas* spp. have a flattened body margin.

Clinical Importance: Heavy burdens can cause loss of production and death. *Argas* spp. act as vectors for *Borrelia anserine* and can cause fowl paralysis. They are uncommon in total-confinement poultry systems.

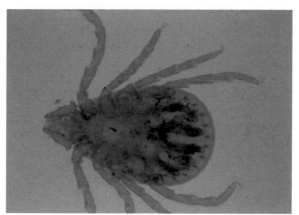

Fig. 4.54. The second segment of the palps of *Haemaphysalis* ticks flares laterally, as seen in this cleared specimen of *H. leporispalustris,* the rabbit tick, which is found in North America. This tick can carry the bacterial agent of tularemia, *Francisella tularensis*. Photo courtesy of Dr. David Baker, School of Veterinary Medicine, Louisiana State University, Baton Rouge, LA.

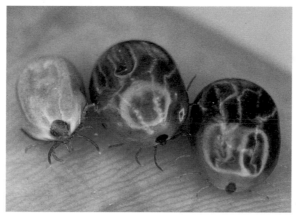

Fig. 4.55. From left to right, engorged *Ixodes, Haemaphysalis,* and *Boophilus* females. Photo courtesy of Dr. Nick Sangster and Ms. Sally Pope, Faculty of Veterinary Science, University of Sydney, Sydney, N.S.W., Australia.

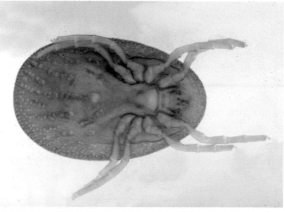

Fig. 4.56. *Argas* sp., the fowl tick, is a soft tick. The ventral location of the mouthparts is clearly seen in this organism. The surface of *Argas* is granulated. Photo courtesy of Dr. Dwight Bowman, College of Veterinary Medicine, Cornell University, Ithaca, NY.

PARASITE: *Otobius megnini* (Figure 4.57)
        Common name: Spinose ear tick.

Taxonomy: Tick (family Argasidae).

Host: Ruminants and horses primarily, also camelids and small animals.

Geographic Distribution: North and South America, Africa, India.

Location on Host: External ear canal.

Life Cycle: Eggs hatch in the environment. Ticks enter the ear of the host and may remain for several months until the nymphal stage is completed. Nymphs leave the host after feeding and molt to the adult stage, which does not feed.

Laboratory Diagnosis: These ticks are easily diagnosed based on host location and recognition of specimens as soft ticks. *Otobius* is covered with short spines, leading to the name spinose ear tick. Hard ticks may also attach in the ears, but they have a distinctive hard, enameled appearance compared to soft ticks like *Otobius*. Also, any adult-stage ticks found in the ears will not be *Otobius*, since spinose ear ticks are parasitic only as larvae and nymphs.

Clinical Importance: Large numbers can cause severe inflammation and rupture the ear drum.

PARASITE: *Ornithodoros* **spp.** (Figure 4.58)
        Common name: Tampan.

Taxonomy: Tick (family Argasidae). *Ornithodoros moubata* is the African tampan; *O. hermsi* is one of the species found in the USA.

Host: Domestic livestock and humans.

Geographic Distribution: Africa, Asia, North and South America.

Location on Host: Various.

Life Cycle: These ticks are often nocturnal and are found in animal or human habitations, including dens, nests, or crevices of buildings.

Laboratory Diagnosis: In contrast to *Argas* spp. ticks, *Ornithodoros* spp. do not have a lateral sutural line and there is no distinct body margin.

Clinical Importance: Large numbers of these soft ticks can cause significant blood loss. *Ornithodoros* transmits endemic relapsing fever in humans. In the USA, *Ornithodoros* ticks are most common in the western and southwestern states.

CLASS INSECTA

Like ticks and mites, insects also belong to the phylum Arthropoda. All insects have bodies composed of three parts: the head, the thorax (which bears the legs), and the abdomen. Adult insects have six legs and some have wings. Life cycles of parasitic insects may be quite simple, in which larval stages are similar in appearance to the adults, or very complex, involving transformation from a wormlike maggot to a pupa and then to the adult. The insects of greatest veterinary importance are the lice, fleas, and flies.

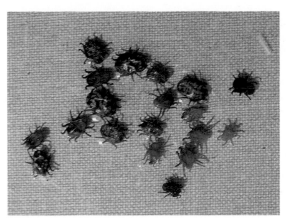

Fig. 4.57. Only larvae and nymphs of *Otobius*, the spinose ear tick, are parasites. They are found clustered in the ears of the host. Unlike the smooth-bodied hard ticks, spines can be seen on the surface of *Otobius* nymphs (not evident at this magnification). Photo courtesy of Dr. Jeffrey F. Williams, Vanson HaloSource, Inc., Redmond, WA.

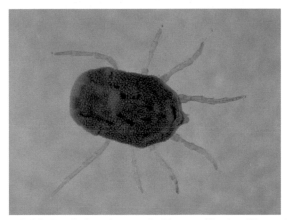

Fig. 4.58. The surface of the soft tick *Ornithodoros* is covered with mammillae (small bumps) and there is no distinct margin to the body.

Lice (Orders Anoplura and Mallophaga)

Lice are wingless, dorsoventrally flattened insects ranging in length from about 1 to 8 mm. They are common ectoparasites of mammals and of birds and infestation may be referred to as "pediculosis." Lice are highly species specific, and the entire life cycle is completed on the host. Immature lice resemble adults but are smaller. Eggs (nits) may be observed attached individually to hair shafts and sometimes as white to yellow masses at the bases of feathers on birds. With close attention, lice can usually be seen with the unaided eye.

Lice are divided into two orders: Mallophaga (chewing or biting lice) and Anoplura (sucking lice). Birds are parasitized only by biting lice, while both biting and sucking lice are found on mammals. The biting lice feed on skin scurf and other organic material on the skin. In contrast, sucking lice feed on blood. Biting lice move rapidly, while sucking lice move more slowly and may be seen head down close to the skin surface or actually feeding. Mallophaga have blunt heads that are wider than the thorax and mandible-like mouth parts and are often a yellow color. Anoplura are generally larger than chewing lice and are gray to dusky red, depending upon the quantity of blood in their intestines. The head of sucking lice is narrower than the thorax and has elongated protrusible piercing mouthparts. While species identification of lice is usually not required in veterinary practice, recognition of an organism as a biting or sucking louse may be helpful when selecting treatment.

Lice on large mammals can also be detected by examining hair coat brushings collected with a stiff-bristled brush. A magnifying lens or dissecting microscope may be useful if lice are very small. Lice may be transferred into saline, mineral or immersion oil, or into Hoyer's solution on a microscope slide with fine forceps, a swab, or a needle moistened with the same material.

PARASITE: *Hematopinus* spp. (Figure 4.59)
Common name: Pig louse, short-nosed cattle louse, cattle tail louse.

Taxonomy: Insect (order Anoplura).

Host: Species important in domestic animals include *H. suis* (pigs), *H. asini* (horses), *H. eurysternus* (short-nosed sucking louse of cattle), and *H. quadripertusus* (tail louse of cattle). Sucking lice are also found on camelids (genus *Microthoracius*).

Geographic Distribution: Worldwide. *Hematopinus quadripertusus* is found primarily in the tropics and subtropics.

Location on Host: *Hematopinus* spp. are often found on the head, neck, and back of the host. *Hematopinus quadripertusus* is usually found around the tail.

Life Cycle: Transmission is by direct contact or fomites. Louse eggs (nits) are glued to the hairs of the host.

Laboratory Diagnosis: Members of this genus are large, about 4–5 mm in length, with the elongated heads typical of the sucking lice.

Clinical Importance: *Hematopinus* infestations can produce alopecia and pruritus, leading to self-inflicted trauma and production losses. Heavy infestations can produce anemia. *Hematopinus suis* is a common and important ectoparasite of swine; *H. eurysternus* is considered the most important cattle louse worldwide. Infestation of horses is uncommon in well-managed stables.

PARASITE: *Linognathus* spp. (Figures 4.60–4.61, 4.68)
Common name: Face louse and foot louse of sheep, long-nosed cattle louse.

Taxonomy: Insect (order Anoplura).

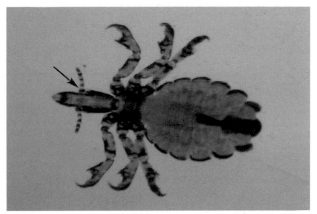

Fig. 4.59. *Hematopinus* spp. have prominent ocular points (*arrow*) and legs of equal size. *Haematopinus suis*, shown here, is the largest louse found on domesticated animals. This dark-colored louse is usually not difficult to identify on the host. Photo courtesy of Dr. Alvin Gajadhar, Centre for Animal Parasitology, CFIA, Saskatoon, Saskatchewan, Canada.

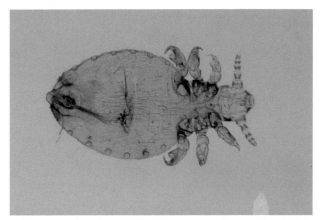

Fig. 4.60. *Linognathus* spp. have no ocular points. Unlike *Haematopinus,* the second and third pairs of legs of these sucking lice are larger than the first pair and end in large claws. The louse shown here is *Linognathus setosus*, the sucking louse of dogs. Members of this genus are usually 2–3 mm in length.

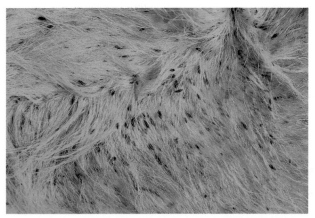

Fig. 4.61. Sucking louse species infesting the skin of a calf. Photo courtesy of Dr. Jeffrey F. Williams, Vanson HaloSource, Inc., Redmond, WA.

Host: *Linognathus pedalis* (ovine foot louse), *L. ovillus* (ovine face louse*)*, *L. vituli* (long-nosed cattle louse*)*, *L. africanus* (bovine African blue louse*)*, *L. setosus* (dogs).

Geographic Distribution: Worldwide.

Location on Host: The face and foot lice of sheep are found primarily in those locations; other species are less restricted in distribution.

Life Cycle: Transmission is by direct contact or fomites.

Laboratory Diagnosis: Detection of lice and eggs on the host by gross observation.

Clinical Importance: As with other lice, infested animals show pruritus and dermatitis, and severe infestations can lead to production losses and anemia.

PARASITE: ***Solenopotes capillatus*** (Figures 4.61–4.62)
              Common name: Little blue cattle louse.

Taxonomy: Insect (order Anoplura).

Host: Cattle.

Geographic Distribution: Worldwide.

Location on Host: Usually found concentrated on face, neck, shoulders, back, and tail.

Life Cycle: The entire life cycle is spent on the host with transmission by direct contact or fomites.

Laboratory Diagnosis: *Solenopotes capillatus* is similar in appearance to *Linognathus*, but *Solenopotes* has tubercles carrying spiracles that project from abdominal segments.

Clinical Importance: Large numbers of lice may cause production loss from dermatitis and anemia.

PARASITE: ***Pediculus* spp., *Phthirus pubis*** (Figures 4.63–4.64)
              Common name: Human head louse, body louse, crab louse.

Taxonomy: Insects (order Anoplura). *Pediculus humanus humanus* is the body louse*;* *Pediculus humanus capita* is the head louse; and *Phthirus pubis* is the pubic or crab louse.

Host: Humans.

Geographic Distribution: Worldwide.

Location on Host: Head lice are found in that region, while body lice live principally in clothing and visit the skin to feed. Crab lice are found in the pubic area or on other coarse body hair.

Life Cycle: Transmission of all human lice infestations is by direct contact or fomites. Head and crab lice glue their eggs to host hair, while body lice deposit their eggs in clothing.

Laboratory Diagnosis: Observation of lice and eggs.

Clinical Importance: Humans are the only hosts of these parasites. Their veterinary importance lies in the occasional detection of a human louse on a pet and resulting confusion about who gave what to whom. In these cases the family pet has lice only because of close contact with infested humans. Human lice do not survive and reproduce on domestic animals.

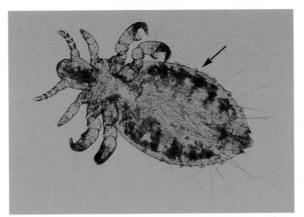

Fig. 4.62. *Solenopotes capillatus*, the little blue cattle louse, is less common than *Linognathus* spp. The projecting tubercles carrying spiracles on the abdominal segments of *Solenopotes* (*arrow*) are helpful in identification of this louse. Photo courtesy of Merial.

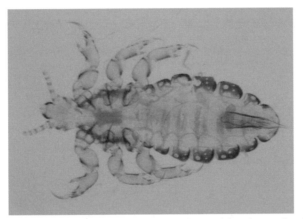

Fig. 4.63. *Pediculus humanus* has well-developed eyes, no ocular points, and three large pairs of legs.

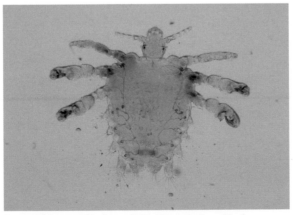

Fig. 4.64. The human crab louse, *Phthirus pubis*, has a distinctive crab-shaped body.

Parasite: Sucking Lice of Laboratory Animals (Figures 4.65–4.66)

Taxonomy: Insect (order Anoplura).

Host: Rodents, rabbits.

Geographic Distribution: Worldwide.

Location on Host: Predilection sites variable, depending on species.

Life Cycle: As with other lice, transmission is by direct contact with an infested animal or fomites.

Laboratory Diagnosis: Detection of eggs and lice on hair and morphological identification of lice.

Clinical Importance: Large numbers of lice may cause loss of condition and possibly anemia.

Parasite: *Bovicola* **spp.** (Figures 4.67–4.72)
            Common name: Biting louse.

Taxonomy: Insect (order Mallophaga).

Host: *Bovicola bovis* (cattle), *B. equi* (horses), *B. ovis* (sheep), *B. caprae* (goats), *B. breviceps* (camelids).

Geographic Distribution: Worldwide.

Location on Host: In general, preferred sites include the neck, shoulder, and back, but lice can spread throughout the body.

Life Cycle: Like the sucking lice, all stages of biting lice are found on the host, and transmission is by direct contact with an infested animal or fomites.

Laboratory Diagnosis: Infested animals should be observed, although *Bovicola* spp. are only a few millimeters in length and may be difficult to see. Hair coat brushings can also be examined with a magnifying glass.

Clinical Importance: These common external parasites cause pruritus and dermatitis and are associated with production losses and secondary infections in heavy infestations.

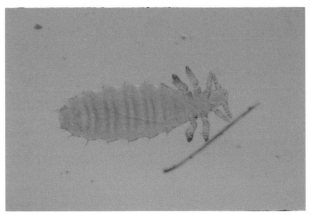

Fig. 4.65. Sucking lice (*Polyplax*) species from a rat. Typical of sucking lice, the head is narrower than the thorax in this specimen.

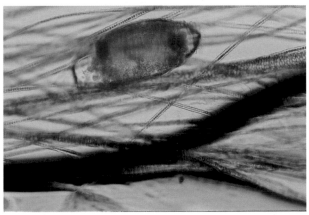

Fig. 4.66. *Polyplax* egg glued to a rat hair. The presence of lice eggs ("nits") on the hairs is helpful in diagnosis of infestation.

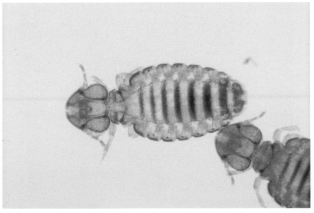

Fig. 4.67. Like other biting lice, the head of *Bovicola* spp. is broader than the thorax. Pictured here is the bovine parasite *Bovicola bovis.* Photo courtesy of Dr. Robert Ridley, College of Veterinary Medicine, Kansas State University, Manhattan, KS.

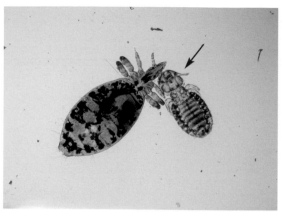

Fig. 4.68. Biting lice of domestic animals are usually smaller than sucking lice. *Bovicola bovis* (*arrow*) is pictured here with one of the bovine sucking lice, *Linognathus*. Photo courtesy of Dr. Robert Ridley, College of Veterinary Medicine, Kansas State University, Manhattan, KS.

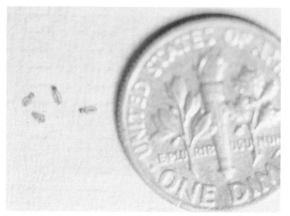

Fig. 4.69. *Bovicola ovis* is a small white or tan louse that can be very difficult to detect on a heavily fleeced sheep. Photo courtesy of Dr. Jeffrey F. Williams, Vanson HaloSource, Inc., Redmond, WA.

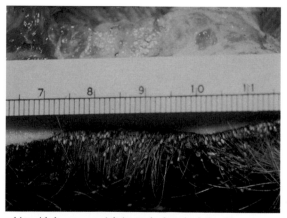

Fig. 4.70. Section of bovine skin with louse eggs (nits) attached to the hairs. Photo courtesy of Dr. Jeffrey F. Williams, Vanson HaloSource, Inc., Redmond, WA.

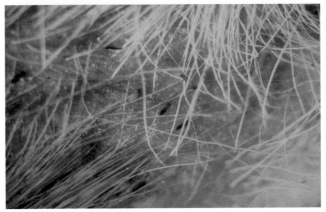

Fig. 4.71. Biting lice (*Bovicola equi*) in the hairs of a horse. Photo courtesy of Dr. Jeffrey F. Williams, Vanson HaloSource, Inc., Redmond, WA.

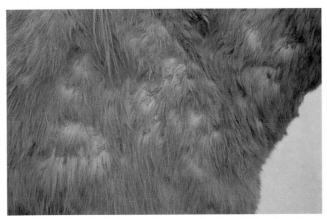

Fig. 4.72. Lesions on the shoulder and neck of a horse with a heavy burden of biting lice. Photo courtesy of Dr. Jeffrey F. Williams, Vanson HaloSource, Inc., Redmond, WA.

PARASITE: *Trichodectes canis* (Figures 4.73–4.75)

Taxonomy: Insect (order Mallophaga).

Host: Dogs and other canids. Cats have their own species of biting louse, *Felicola subrostratus*.

Geographic Distribution: Worldwide. Another species of biting louse, *Heterodoxus spinigera,* may also be found on dogs in tropical and subtropical areas.

Location on Host: Predilection sites for *T. canis* are the head, neck, and tail, but lice will be found throughout the hair coat in heavy infestations.

Life Cycle: Transmission is by direct contact or fomites. Louse eggs are glued to host hairs.

Laboratory Diagnosis: Recovery and identification of lice. *Felicola* is the only louse infesting cats, although infestations on cats may be difficult to diagnose because of the effective grooming habits of the host. Dogs can be infested with the biting lice *Trichodectes* and *Heterodoxus,* as well as the sucking louse, *Linognathus setosus.*

Clinical Importance: Large infestations of lice cause pruritus and poor hair condition. *Trichodectes* is the most common dog louse seen in the USA and can act as an intermediate host for the tapeworm *Dipylidium caninum.*

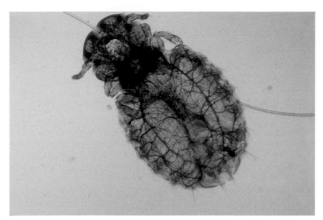

Fig. 4.73. *Trichodectes canis* is the canine biting louse.

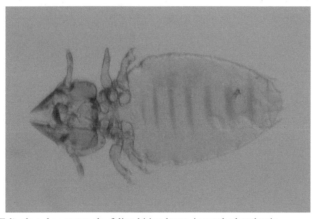

Fig. 4.74. The head of *Felicola subrostratus,* the feline biting louse, is notched at the tip.

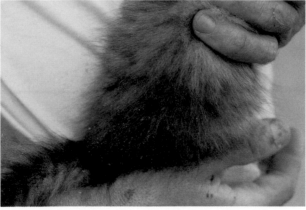

Fig. 4.75. White louse eggs (nits) can be seen attached to the hairs of this infested kitten. Photo courtesy of Dr. Jeffrey F. Williams, Vanson HaloSource, Inc., Redmond, WA.

PARASITE: Avian Lice (Figures 4.76–4.78)

Taxonomy: Insects (order Mallophaga).

Host: Lice are common external parasites of birds, and multiple louse species may be found occupying different niches on the same host species. All avian lice are biting lice.

Geographic Distribution: Worldwide.

Location on Host: Lice can be found on all areas of birds, with different species showing specific predilection sites.

Life Cycle: Similar to other lice; the entire life cycle is spent on the host, and transmission is by direct contact or fomites.

Laboratory Diagnosis: Detection of lice and eggs on the host with morphologic identification of lice.

Clinical Importance: Heavy infestations may cause loss of condition. Sick or malnourished birds often carry large numbers of lice.

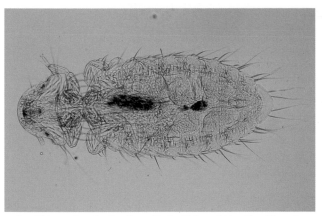

Fig. 4.76. There are more than 700 species of avian lice, all of which are biting lice. They show a variety of body shapes. Shown here is *Menopon gallinae*, the shaft louse of chickens.

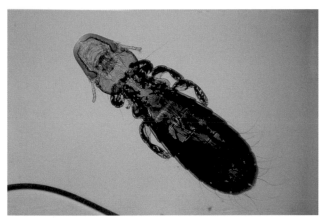

Fig. 4.77. *Lipeurus caponis,* the wing louse of poultry.

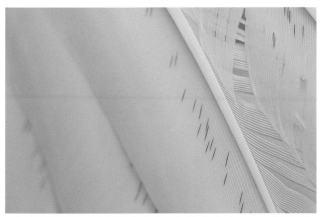

Fig. 4.78. *Columbicula columbae*, the slender pigeon louse, on the flight feathers of a pigeon. Photo courtesy of Dr. Jeffrey F. Williams, Vanson HaloSource, Inc., Redmond, WA.

Parasite: *Gliricola porcelli* (Figure 4.79)

Common name: Slender guinea pig louse.

Taxonomy: Insect (order Mallophaga).

Host: *Gliricola porcelli* is the most common louse of guinea pigs. Two other species of biting lice, *Gyropus ovalis* and *Trimenopon jenningsi*, are also found on guinea pigs.

Geographic Distribution: Worldwide.

Location on Host: *Gliricola procelli* prefers the fine hair around the back legs and anus, whereas *Gyropus ovalis* is found around the head and face.

Life Cycle: Transmission is by direct contact.

Laboratory Diagnosis: Detection and identification of lice and eggs. *Gyropus ovalis* is a broader louse than *Giricola* and has a wide head. Eggs of *G. ovalis* can be found most easily around the back of the ears. *Trimenopon jenningsi* is a dark brown louse that is less common than the other 2 species.

Clinical Importance: Light infestations are usually asymptomatic. Heavier infestations may be associated with hair loss, unthriftiness, and pruritus, especially at the back of the ears. Louse infestation may not be evident until the death of the host, when lice move up to the hair tips as the body temperature declines.

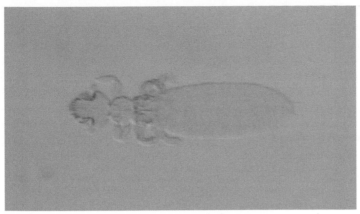

Fig. 4.79. *Gliricola porcelli,* one of three species of biting louse infecting guinea pigs.

Fleas (Order Siphonaptera)

Fleas are laterally compressed, wingless insects, typically medium to dark brown in color. Unlike many insects, they do not demonstrate clear delineations between body regions (head, thorax, and abdomen). The sucking mouthparts are usually seen protruding from the ventral aspect of the head. The three pairs of legs originate on the thorax. The enlarged third pair of legs facilitates the incredible jumping potential of these insects. In veterinary medicine, fleas are most often encountered on dogs and cats; however, they also live on a variety of other animals, including birds. Fleas are more likely than lice to move onto a different host species if the preferred host is unavailable, although they may leave after obtaining a blood meal. The adult flea is the only parasitic stage of the life cycle. The egg, larva, and pupa are found in the environment.

Fleas can be seen with the naked eye. They are most easily collected from the host by using a quick-acting insecticide and then removing individual fleas from the hair coat or combing them out with a flea comb. On birds, fleas may be attached to the unfeathered portions of the host and can be removed with forceps. Fleas should be placed in 70% ethanol for fixation and storage. They may be cleared in 5% potassium hydroxide or mounted in Hoyer's solution to allow visualization of reproductive structures used in identification. The presence of combs on the cheek (genal comb) or at the back of the first thoracic segment (pronotal comb), the shape of the head, and host preference are important characteristics used in identification. Figure 4.80 is a key for identification of some common species in North America. In many cases, a specialist is required for specific identification. When submitting fleas for identification, it is best to submit as many individuals as possible to ensure that both sexes are represented and that structures damaged on one individual are still intact on another.

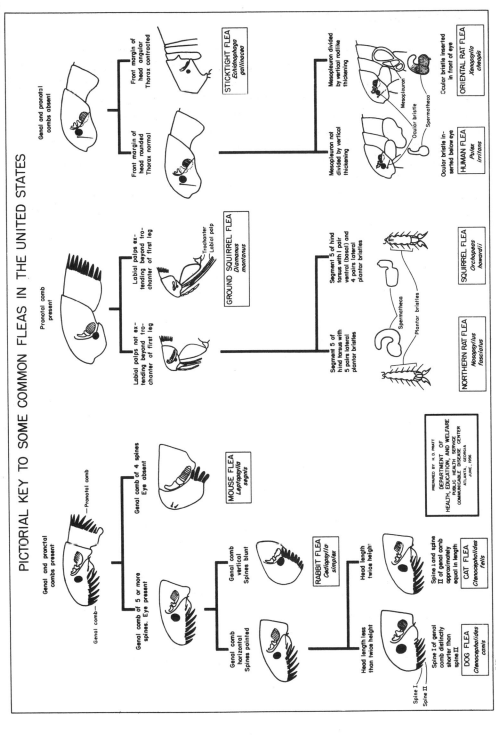

Fig. 4.80. Key to common flea species in the USA. Courtesy of US Public Health Service, CDC.

Parasite: *Ctenocephalides felis felis* (Figures 4.81–4.84)
     Common name: Cat flea.

Taxonomy: Insect (order Siphonaptera). A similar species, *Ctenocephalides canis,* also occurs but is less common than *C. felis felis* on both dogs and cats.

Host: Cats, dogs, ferrets. Occasionally populations may adapt to living on confined animals, such as goats or calves in a barn.

Geographic Distribution: Worldwide. *Ctenocephalides* is the most common flea of dogs and cats.

Location on Host: Fleas can be found throughout the hair coat, but predilection sites include the tail head, neck, and flanks.

Life Cycle: Adults cat fleas seldom leave the host. Females deposit eggs that fall off the host and hatch in the environment. Flea larvae feed on organic debris and adult flea feces and pupate in the environment. Adults are stimulated to emerge from the pupa by vibration and mechanical compression. Under optimum conditions, the life cycle can be completed in about 2 weeks.

Laboratory Diagnosis: Cat fleas have both pronotal and genal combs.

Size:	Adult female	approx. 2.5 mm in length
	Adult male	approx. 1 mm in length
	Larva	approx. 5 mm in length

Clinical Importance: Low levels of flea infestation may be mildly pruritic. Large flea populations can produce severe pruritus, alopecia, and anemia. Animals that develop flea-bite hypersensitivity may suffer severe dermatologic disease even when flea numbers are very low.

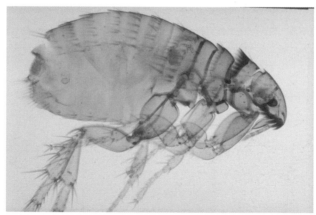

Fig. 4.81. Female *Ctenocephalides felis felis*. The cat flea is the most common flea found on both dogs and cats. It is difficult to differentiate from the less common *Ctenocephalides canis*. Characteristics helpful in identifying this genus are the genal and pronotal combs. Photo courtesy of Dr. Byron Blagburn, College of Veterinary Medicine, Auburn University, Auburn, AL.

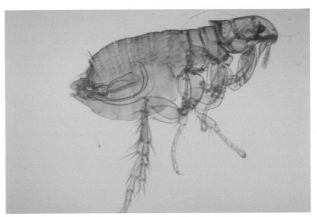

Fig. 4.82. Male *Ctenocephalides felis felis*. Male cat fleas are smaller than females. Photo courtesy of Dr. Byron Blagburn, College of Veterinary Medicine, Auburn University, Auburn, AL.

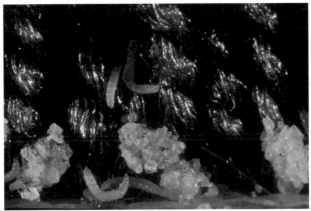

Fig. 4.83. *Ctenocephalides* spp. eggs are about 0.5 mm long. Larvae and pupae (covered with sand grains) of the cat flea are shown in this figure. The surface of the pupa is sticky and becomes camouflaged with environmental debris. Photo courtesy of Dr. Byron Blagburn, College of Veterinary Medicine, Auburn University, Auburn, AL.

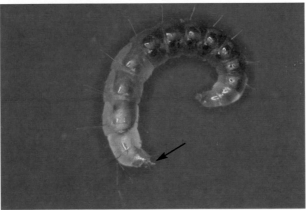

Fig. 4.84. Pet owners may find larvae of the cat flea, *C. felis felis*, in their homes and present them for identification. Mature larvae are about 5 mm long. The two "anal struts" projecting from the posterior end of the body (*arrow*) are distinctive. Photo courtesy of Dr. Byron Blagburn, College of Veterinary Medicine, Auburn University, Auburn, AL.

PARASITE: *Pulex irritans* (Figure 4.85)
                    Common name: Human flea.

Taxonomy: Insect (order Siphonaptera). *P. simulans* is a closely related species found on dogs and cats in the New World.

Host: Humans, pigs, dogs, cats.

Geographic Distribution: Worldwide.

Location on Host: General distribution on the host.

Life Cycle: Like *Ctenocephalides felis felis,* only adults are found on the host; other stages are present in the environment.

Laboratory Diagnosis: Identification of adult fleas. *Pulex irritans* has no genal or pronotal combs and possesses an ocular bristle below the eye.

Clinical Importance: Worldwide, *Pulex irritans* is found more often on swine than on humans or cats and dogs. Heavy flea infestations can produce intense irritation and pruritus. *Pulex irritans* is uncommon in North America, although it has been recorded from most states in the United States. *Pulex* spp. can serve as a vector of *Yersinia pestis*, the bubonic plague bacillus, and *Rickettsia typhi*, the agent of murine typhus.

PARASITE: **Fleas of Rodents and Rabbits** (Figures 4.86–4.87)

Taxonomy: Insects (order Siphonaptera).

Host: A variety of species parasitize rodents and rabbits, including *Xenopsylla cheopsis* (oriental rat flea), an important vector of bubonic plague. *Xenopsylla cheopsis* will also readily feed on dogs, cats, humans, and other animals when normal rodent hosts are unavailable.

Geographic Distribution: Worldwide.

Location on Host: General distribution on the host. *Spilopsyllus cuniculi,* a flea of rabbits, attaches to the skin in the ears for long periods of time in a manner similar to *Echidnophaga gallinacea,* the sticktight flea of birds (see below).

Life Cycle: Similar to other fleas. Some species of rodent flea only visit the host to feed, unlike the common cat flea, which is resident on the host as an adult.

Laboratory Diagnosis: Rodent and rabbit fleas are identified based on morphologic characteristics.

Clinical Importance: *Xenopsylla cheopsis* and some other rodent fleas are vectors of bubonic plague, caused by *Yersinia pestis*, and murine typhus, caused by *Rickettsia typhi.* Because the bacteria interfere with normal flea feeding, fleas rapidly move from host to host, spreading infection. Other rodent fleas can transmit tapeworms, trypanosomes, and myxomatosis to rabbits.

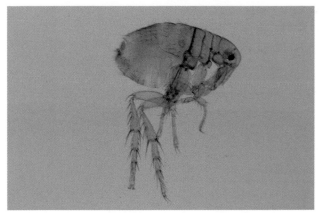

Fig. 4.85. The human flea, *Pulex irritans,* is less common on people in industrialized countries. It may also be found on companion animals and pigs. The absence of genal and pronotal combs and location of the ocular bristle are helpful in identification.

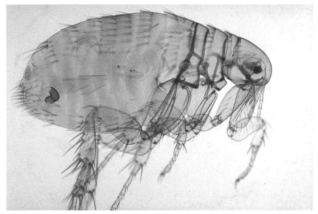

Fig. 4.86. *Xenopsylla cheopsis*, the oriental rat flea. Fleas belonging to several genera are found on rodents and rabbits. Photo courtesy of Dr. Byron Blagburn, College of Veterinary Medicine, Auburn University, Auburn, AL.

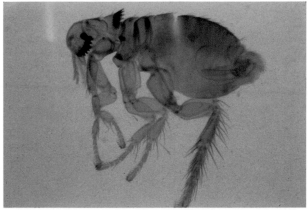

Fig. 4.87. *Cediopsylla simplex,* a rabbit flea. Photo courtesy of Dr. David Baker, School of Veterinary Medicine, Louisiana State University, Baton Rouge, LA.

PARASITE: *Echidnophaga gallinacea, Ceratophyllus* **spp.** (Figure 4.88)
Common name: Sticktight flea, European chicken flea.

Taxonomy: Insects (order Siphonaptera).

Host: *Echidnophaga gallinacea,* the sticktight flea, is found on poultry, wild birds, and occasionally on dogs, cats, and other animals. *Ceratophyllus* spp. are parasites of wild and domestic birds, especially chickens.

Geographic Distribution: Worldwide. *Echidnophaga* is found primarily in tropical and subtropical regions of the New World.

Location on Host: The sticktight flea is usually found on nonfeathered skin on the head, comb, and wattles of poultry.

Life Cycle: The life cycle of poultry fleas is similar to other fleas, but female *Echidnophaga* attach permanently to the head of the host. Eggs are deposited either onto the ground or into the sore created at the attachment site.

Laboratory Diagnosis: Identification of adult fleas. Female *Echidnophaga* can be identified by their location and attachment. This species also lacks genal and pronotal combs and has a sharply angled head. *Ceratophyllus* has a pronotal comb.

Size:	Female *Echidnophaga*	approx. 2 mm in length
	Ceratophyllus	approx. 4 mm in length

Clinical Importance: Sticktight fleas may cause severe irritation by their attachment to birds and other hosts. Heavy infestations can produce anemia. In wild birds, attachment near the eyes may lead to blindness and death. Heavy infestations of *Ceratophyllus* have been associated with anemia, restlessness, and decreased production.

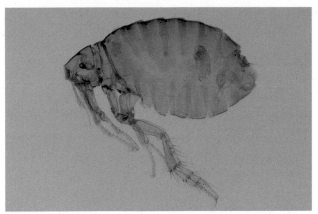

Fig. 4.88. *Echidnophaga gallinacea*, the sticktight flea, has no combs and a sharply angled head.

Flies (Order Diptera)

Flies belong to the order Diptera and some species are parasites in the adult or larval stage. Parasitic adult flies are usually blood feeders. Larval flies parasitizing animals are referred to as either "bots" ("grubs" and "warbles" are synonymous terms) or "maggots." Bots are obligate parasites, found in specific internal locations in the host. Mature bot larvae are barrel shaped and may have rows of spines on the body. Maggots are fly larvae associated with "fly strike," or "fly blow." In most cases they are opportunistic parasites. Adult flies attracted to wounds or hair stained with feces or blood lay their eggs on the animal, and larvae feed on debris and necrotic tissue. Maggots are more elongated than bots and are narrower at the anterior than at the posterior end. They are usually present on the surface of the body in conjunction with wounds or hair soiled with feces, urine, blood, or other organic material. A specialist can identify the genus of a bot or maggot by examining the pattern of the spiracular plates surrounding the breathing holes (spiracles) on the posterior end of the larva.

PARASITE: *Cuterebra* spp. (Figures 4.89–4.91)
     Common name: Rodent bot fly.

Taxonomy: Insect (order Diptera).

Host: Rodents and rabbits are the principal hosts. Dogs, cats, and rarely humans may also be infected.

Geographic Distribution: Western Hemisphere.

Location on Host: Larvae are found in subcutaneous cysts in various locations. In dogs and cats they are seen most often on the head and neck.

Life Cycle: Adult flies lay eggs around rodent holes or trails. Larvae crawl onto animals and enter through facial orifices. Following migration to subcutaneous sites, the *Cuterebra* larva forms a visible nodule with an external breathing hole. After completing development, the larva leaves the host through the breathing hole and pupates on the ground.

Laboratory Diagnosis: *Cuterebra* larvae can usually be identified by location on the host. Specific identification is performed by examination of larval spiracular plates.

Clinical Importance: The presence of one or two bots in both the normal rodent hosts or dogs and cats is usually not associated with clinical problems, although secondary bacterial infections may develop. In dogs and cats abnormal migration to the nervous system or other tissues occasionally occurs and produces disease.

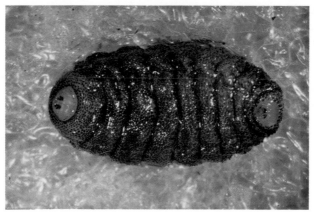

Fig. 4.89. *Cuterebra* larvae are about 2.5 cm in length and dark colored when fully developed. Photo courtesy of Dr. Philip Scholl, Agricultural Research Service, US Department of Agriculture, University of Nebraska, Lincoln, NE.

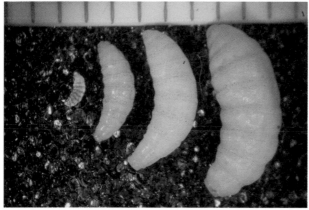

Fig. 4.90. Veterinary practitioners occasionally remove young *Cuterebra* larvae from animals and, because of their small size and white color, may have difficulty recognizing them as *Cuterebra*. Starting at the left, this Fig. shows larvae at 6, 8, 10, and 13 days after infestation of the host. Photo courtesy of Dr. Philip Scholl, Agricultural Research Service, US Department of Agriculture, University of Nebraska, Lincoln, NE.

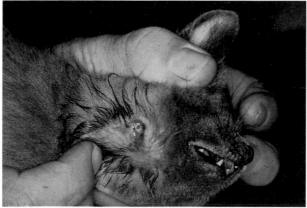

Fig. 4.91. This lesion caused by *Cuterebra* in a cat has become secondarily infected. The posterior end of the bot with its brown spiracular plates is visible. Photo courtesy of Dr. Jeffrey F. Williams, Vanson HaloSource, Inc., Redmond, WA.

PARASITE: *Gastrophilus* **spp.** (Figures 4.92–4.94)
    Common name: Stomach bot.

Taxonomy: Insect (order Diptera). Species include *G. intestinalis, G. nasalis,* and *G. haemorrhoidalis.*

Host: Horses and other equids.

Geographic Distribution: Worldwide.

Location on Host: Equine stomach.

Life Cycle: Adult flies deposit eggs on the legs or face of horses. After hatching, larvae enter through the mouth and spend a period of development on the tongue and gums before moving to the stomach. After a period of 8–11 months in the stomach, bots pass out in the feces and pupate on the ground.

Laboratory Diagnosis: Bots are usually identified by presence in the stomach at necropsy, but they may also be seen in the feces at different stages of development following treatment of the host with macrolide anthelmintics. They can be recognized as bots by their barrel shape and rows of spines.

Clinical Importance: Horses appear to tolerate small to moderate burdens of bots. Large numbers may cause gastric ulceration. In rare instances, humans in close contact with horses are infested and develop a transient dermatitis usually occurring on the face.

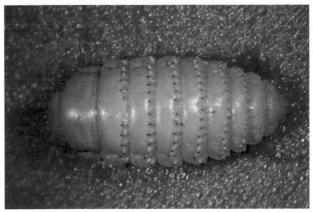

Fig. 4.92. Equine stomach bot, *Gastrophilus*. Species can be distinguished based on patterns of spines on the body, but species identification is unnecessary for control and treatment of the parasite. Photo courtesy of Dr. Philip Scholl, Agricultural Research Service, US Department of Agriculture, University of Nebraska, Lincoln, NE.

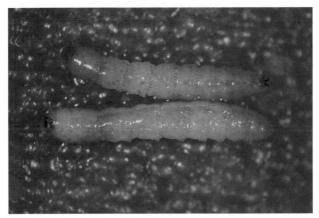

Fig. 4.93. Second-instar *Gastrophilus* larvae. Following treatment with macrolide anthelmintics or other effective drugs, young *Gastrophilus* larvae may also be present in manure. Although the less mature larvae lack the barrel shape of mature bots, they still show the distinctive rows of spines around each segment. Photo courtesy of Dr. Philip Scholl, Agricultural Research Service, US Department of Agriculture, University of Nebraska, Lincoln, NE.

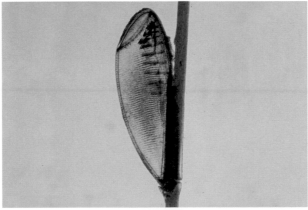

Fig. 4.94. The eggs of *Gastrophilus intestinalis*, the most common equine bot species, can be seen attached to the hairs of the forelegs. Photo courtesy of Dr. Jeffrey F. Williams, Vanson HaloSource, Inc., Redmond, WA.

PARASITE: *Hypoderma bovis, H. lineatum* (Figures 4.95–4.97)
Common name: Cattle grub, ox warble.

Taxonomy: Insect (order Diptera).

Host: Cattle are the normal hosts; horses and goats are occasionally infested. Other species of *Hypoderma* parasitize deer and reindeer, and *Przhevalskiana silenus* is a similar parasite of goats in the Mediterranean region.

Geographic Distribution: North America, Europe, Asia.

Location on Host: Visible nodules with an external opening appear on the backs of infested animals.

Life Cycle: Adult flies deposit eggs on cattle. After hatching, larvae penetrate through the skin and migrate to sites either along the esophagus or in the tissue surrounding the spinal cord. After a period of development lasting several months, the larvae migrate to the host's back and form subcutaneous nodules with a breathing hole. After several more months of development, larvae emerge and pupate on the ground and adult flies are formed.

Laboratory Diagnosis: Diagnosis can usually be made based on parasite location in the host and history.

Clinical Importance: Damage from *Hypoderma* comes from several sources. Adult fly activity associated with oviposition worries cattle and may interfere with grazing; migrating larvae cause necrotic tracks in muscle tissue and the hide is damaged for leather production. In addition, if larvae die while along the esophagus or spinal cord, serious inflammatory reactions can lead to bloat or paralysis.

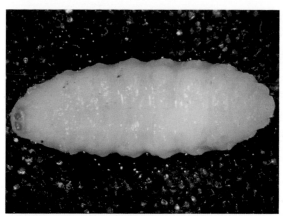

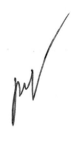

Fig. 4.95. Early third-instar cattle grub, *Hypoderma lineatum*. Grubs or warbles can be distinguished from fly maggots by their barrel-shaped bodies and typical location in the host. Photo courtesy of Dr. Philip Scholl, Agricultural Research Service, US Department of Agriculture, University of Nebraska, Lincoln, NE.

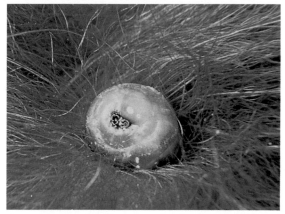

Fig. 4.96. *Hypoderma* sp. grub emerging from its subcutaneous location on the back of the bovine host. Photo courtesy of Dr. Philip Scholl, Agricultural Research Service, US Department of Agriculture, University of Nebraska, Lincoln, NE, and Dr. Jerry Weintraub, Agriculture Canada, Lethbridge, Alberta, Canada.

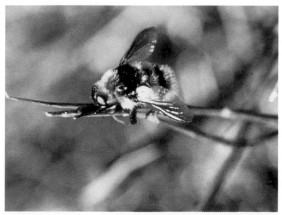

Fig. 4.97. The hairy body of adult warble (bot) flies makes them look more like bees than flies. The presence of adult warble flies, like this *Hypoderma bovis*, is distressing to potential hosts, which will actively try to avoid the flies. Photo courtesy of Dr. Philip Scholl, Agricultural Research Service, US Department of Agriculture, University of Nebraska, Lincoln, NE, and Dr. Jerry Weintraub, Agriculture Canada, Lethbridge, Alberta, Canada.

253

PARASITE: *Oestrus ovis, Rhinoestrus* spp. (Figure 4.98)
Common name: Sheep nasal bot.

Taxonomy: Insects (order Diptera).

Host: *Oestrus ovis* larvae are found in sheep and goats. *Rhinoestrus* larvae are found in horses. Other species parasitize deer and camels (e.g., *Cephalopina titillator*).

Geographic Distribution: *Oestrus ovis* is found worldwide. *Rhinoestrus* infestation occurs in Africa, Europe, and Asia.

Location on Host: Nasal passages and sinuses.

Life Cycle: Adult female flies deposit larvae in or near the nasal passages. Larvae develop in nasal passages and sinuses. When development is complete, they fall out of the nose and pupate on the ground.

Laboratory Diagnosis: Nasal bots are not usually presented for identification because of their location, but they are sometimes found by owners in water troughs or on the ground after they exit the host. Specific identification is made by examination of the spiracular plates.

Clinical Importance: Although infested animals show increased levels of nasal discharge, small or moderate numbers of bots are usually well tolerated. Sheep will attempt to avoid ovipositing female flies by keeping their muzzles near the ground or under available shelter (buildings, cars, one another, etc.). Bots occasionally wander to abnormal sites, where they may cause serious disease.

PARASITE: *Dermatobia hominis* (Figure 4.99)
Common name: Human bot fly.

Taxonomy: Insect (order Diptera).

Host: Cattle, humans, dogs, other domestic and wild animals.

Geographic Distribution: Central and South America.

Location on Host: Various subcutaneous sites.

Life Cycle: Adult female *Dermatobia* glue clusters of eggs to various muscid flies and mosquitoes. When these organisms visit a host, the *Dermatobia* larvae are deposited and enter the subcutaneous tissue, where each larva develops in a nodule with a hole in the skin through which respiration occurs. Larvae leave the host to pupate.

Laboratory Diagnosis: Identification of larvae is based on shape and pattern of the spiracles.

Clinical Importance: This species is best known as a human parasite, although it is primarily a pest of cattle.

PARASITE: **Louse Flies, Including** *Melophagus ovinus* (Figures 4.100–4.101)
Common name: Sheep ked, louse fly.

Taxonomy: Insects (order Diptera).

Host: Sheep and goats are parasitized by *Melophagus ovinus*, the sheep ked. Louse flies may be found on a variety of animals. Examples include *Hippobosca variegata* on horses, cattle, and camels; *Lipoptena* spp. on deer; *Hippobosca longipennis* on dogs; and *Pseudolynchia* spp. on birds.

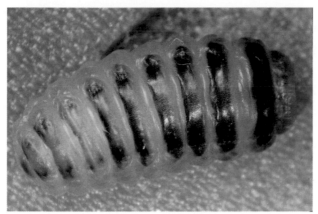

Fig. 4.98. Ovine nasal bot, *Oestrus ovis*. These bots are occasionally seen by producers when they leave the small ruminant host to pupate or following treatment. Photo courtesy of Dr. Philip Scholl, Agricultural Research Service, US Department of Agriculture, University of Nebraska, Lincoln, NE.

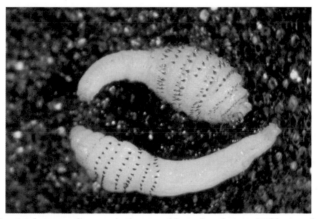

Fig. 4.99. *Dermatobia hominis* bots are often seen in the second-instar larval stage. At this stage they have a distinctive narrow, spineless posterior end that becomes less prominent as they continue development. Photo courtesy of Dr. Philip Scholl, Agricultural Research Service, US Department of Agriculture, University of Nebraska, Lincoln, NE.

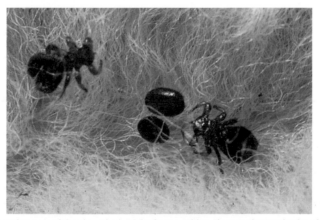

Fig. 4.100. Adult and pupal stages of the sheep ked, *Melophagus*. Although sometimes mistaken for ticks, these organisms are insects with six legs and three main body parts. Ked excrement, which resembles flea feces, can also be found on the host and is helpful in diagnosis. Photo courtesy of Dr. Jeffrey F. Williams, Vanson HaloSource, Inc., Redmond, WA.

Geographic Distribution: Worldwide, although in North America only the sheep ked and the pigeon fly *(Pseudolynchia)* are found on domestic animals.

Location on Host: Various.

Life Cycle: In some species winged adult flies are temporary parasites while feeding; in others they lose their wings after finding a host and become permanent parasites. The sheep ked, *Melophagus,* has no functional wings and is transmitted only by direct contact of hosts. Adult female sheep keds deposit larvae that pupate immediately on the skin of the host.

Laboratory Diagnosis: Identification is based on adult flies. Hippoboscid flies generally have a rather flat, leathery appearance compared to other flies. Ked feces, which resemble flea feces, may be found on the host.

Clinical Importance: Sheep keds can cause significant damage to the skin, making it unsuitable for leather production, and can also reduce the value of the sheep fleece. Biting activity of flies causes pain and irritation.

PARASITE: Fly Strike or Blow Flies (Figures 4.102–4.103)

Taxonomy: Insects (order Diptera). Many of the maggots causing fly strike belong to the families Calliphoridae (blow flies) and Sarcophagidae (flesh flies).

Host: Various, not host specific.

Geographic Distribution: Worldwide.

Location on Host: Various, wherever there is blood or other body secretion that attracts female flies.

Life Cycle: Larvae of most of the flies in this group are not obligatory parasites. Adults are attracted by the odors of decaying organic material and deposit their eggs on carrion. Wounds or skin on animals soiled with blood or feces may also attract the flies. Larvae feed primarily on necrotic material, and when development is completed, they leave the host and pupate in the environment.

Laboratory Diagnosis: Recognition of maggots on animals is sufficient for diagnosis of fly strike. Specific identification of fly larvae requires examination of larval spiracles.

Clinical Importance: "Flyblown" animals can be seriously affected by fly larvae. The presence of large numbers of maggots may produce tissue destruction, toxemia, and even death.

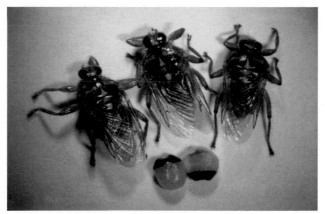

Fig. 4.101. Typical hippoboscid louse flies showing the flattened appearance of the body with relatively large legs and wings. Photo courtesy of Dr. Alvin Gajadhar, Centre for Animal Parasitology, CFIA, Saskatoon, Saskatchewan, Canada.

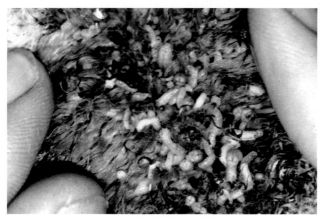

Fig. 4.102. A case of ovine "fly strike," or "fly blow," in which an animal has become infested with fly maggots. In most cases these flies are not true parasites and would be equally attracted to carrion. Sheep are particularly susceptible to fly strike in warm weather if wool is persistently wet or becomes soiled with blood or feces. Photo courtesy of Dr. Dwight Bowman, College of Veterinary Medicine, Cornell University, Ithaca, NY.

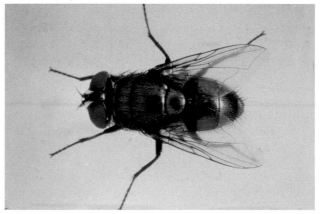

Fig. 4.103. *Lucilia* spp. is one of the genera of blow flies that cause facultative myiasis (fly strike). Blow flies are typically metallic blue, green, or bronze in color. *Lucilia* spp. infestations of sheep are a source of significant economic loss to the Australian sheep industry. Photo courtesy of Dr. Nick Sangster and Ms. Sally Pope, Faculty of Veterinary Science, University of Sydney, Sydney, NSW, Australia.

PARASITE: *Cochliomyia hominivorax, Chrysomya bezziana* (Figures 4.104–4.105)
> Common name: Screwworm.

Taxonomy: Insects (order Diptera). Screwworms belong to the blow fly family (Calliphoridae). Several species of sarcophagid flies are also obligatory parasites but are of less importance.

Host: Wild and domestic animals, humans.

Geographic Distribution: *Cochliomyia hominivorax,* the New World screwworm, is found in South America. The Old World screwworm, *Chrysomya bezziana*, occurs in Africa, India, and Southeast Asia.

Location on Host: Various, often on body openings or the edges of wounds.

Life Cycle: Adult female flies deposit eggs on the host. Larvae feed invasively on living tissue. Following completion of development, larvae fall to the ground and pupate. Adults emerge and mate. The entire life cycle can be completed in as little as 24 days.

Laboratory Diagnosis: Examination of larval spiracles is important for larval identification. The larvae also have two posterior tracheal trunks, which look like dark lines extending anteriorly from the posterior end. Although screwworm has been eradicated from the USA, reintroduction is possible. If screwworm infestation is suspected, larvae should be collected in 70% alcohol and submitted to federal or state veterinarians for identification.

Clinical Importance: Screwworm infestation is a serious disease that can rapidly lead to the death of the host. The parasite was eradicated from the USA in the 1960s through a sterile-male release program. This program has now been successful in removing the fly from Mexico and Central America, with only occasional outbreaks still reported.

PARASITE: **Biting Flies** (Figures 4.106–4.113)
> Common name: Horse fly, deer fly, mosquito, black fly, sand fly, tsetse fly, horn fly, stable fly, midge, etc.

Taxonomy: Insects (order Diptera). Biting flies belong to many families within the order.

Host: Domestic and wild animals and humans.

Geographic Distribution: Worldwide.

Location on Host: Various, although many biting flies have predilection sites.

Life Cycle: Like other Diptera, biting flies lay eggs that hatch into larvae. Pupation follows a period of larval development, followed by the emergence of adult flies. In some biting fly species, like the mosquito, only the females are blood feeders. In other species, adults of both sexes feed on blood.

Laboratory Diagnosis: Although detailed descriptions of biting flies are not within the scope of this book, some generalizations can be made that allow basic identification (see figures).

Clinical Importance: Biting flies have enormous importance in veterinary medicine because of their role as disease vectors. Mosquitoes alone transmit important protozoan, helminth, and viral diseases of animals and humans. In addition, the activity of biting flies causes irritation, and their bites can lead to allergic dermatitis and, in some cases of massive fly attacks, even toxemia and death.

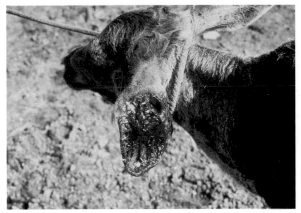

Fig. 4.104. Screwworm infestation on the ear of a calf. If untreated these infestations are often fatal. Photo courtesy of Dr. Donald B. Thomas, USDA Subtropical Agriculture Research Laboratory, Weslaco, TX.

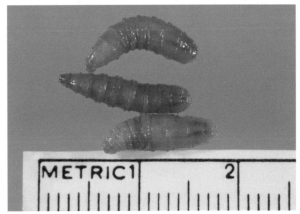

Fig. 4.105. Screwworm maggots. If screwworm infestation is suspected in the USA, larvae should be submitted in 70% alcohol to state or federal veterinarians.

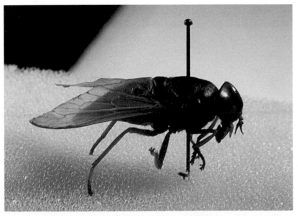

Fig. 4.106. Tabanid flies. These large biting flies with big eyes are familiar worldwide. Horse flies may reach 2.5 cm in length. Deer flies, *Chrysops*, also belong to this group. Deer flies are smaller and have distinct bands on their wings; horse flies have unmarked or diffusely marked wings. This Fig. shows a large *Tabanus* sp. horse fly. Photo courtesy of Dr. Jeffrey F. Williams, Vanson HaloSource, Inc., Redmond, WA.

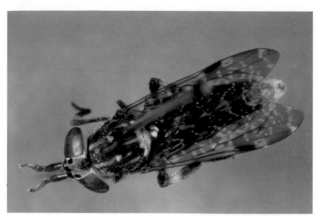

Fig. 4.107. Horse fly from the genus *Haematopota*, which is uncommon in North America. Photo courtesy of Dr. Alvin Gajadhar, Centre for Animal Parasitology, CFIA, Saskatoon, Saskatchewan, Canada.

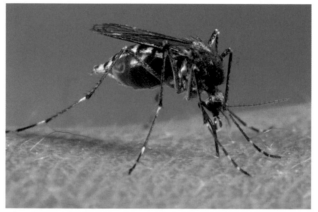

Fig. 4.108. Most people in the world need little description of mosquitoes since they are common in so many regions. Mosquitoes belong to a number of genera and their larvae develop in water. These delicate flies with long legs have mouthparts that are at least twice as long as the head. Photo from Agricultural Research Service, US Department of Agriculture.

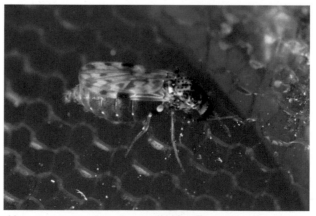

Fig. 4.109. *Culicoides* (midges or no-see-ums) are very small biting flies (rarely larger than 2 mm) with patterned wings. Species are found worldwide. Photo from Agricultural Research Service, US Department of Agriculture.

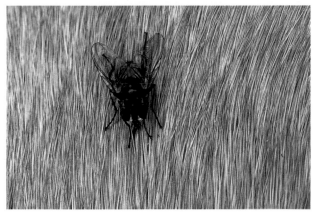

Fig. 4.110. *Stomoxys calcitrans,* the common stable fly. These flies are very similar in appearance to the house fly, *Musca domestica*, but when at rest in the environment their mouthparts project from the head at a right angle, which can be seen without magnification. Photo courtesy of Merial.

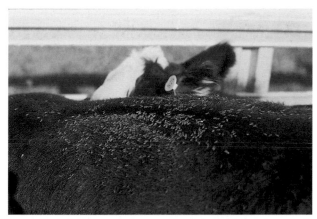

Fig. 4.111. Horn flies, *Haematobia irritans,* are a major pest of cattle in North America and other parts of the world. Horn flies can be identified by their behavior. They cluster on the dorsum of the host, heads pointing toward the ground. If disturbed, they fly a short distance into the air and rapidly settle on the host again. Photo courtesy of Dr. Jeffrey F. Williams, Vanson HaloSource, Inc., Redmond, WA.

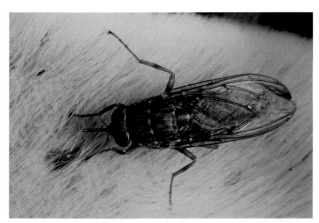

Fig. 4.112. *Glossina*, the tsetse fly, is the vector of trypanosomiasis in domestic animals and humans in Africa. Species of this fly reach up to 14 mm in length. Like stable flies, the mouthparts of the fly project forward from the head, but the wings of tsetse flies lie across the back like scissors. Photo courtesy of Dr. Andrew Peregrine, Ontario Veterinary College, University of Guelph, Guelph, Ontario, Canada.

Other Insects

PARASITE: *Cimex* **spp.** (Figure 4.114)
          Common name: Bedbug.

Taxonomy: Insect (order Hemiptera).

Host: Humans and domestic animals. Other members of the genus parasitize birds and bats.

Geographic Distribution: Worldwide.

Location on Host: Bedbugs do not have specific predilection sites on the host.

Life Cycle: Bedbugs visit the host only at night to feed and spend daylight hours in cracks and crevices in human or animal environments. Eggs are laid in the environment.

Laboratory Diagnosis: Identification of dorsoventrally flattened insects. Adults are 5–7 mm in length. In human infestations, bedbug feces may be seen in the bed.

Clinical Importance: Bedbugs are most important as human parasites, but they will also attack domestic animals. In the USA, bedbugs have recently become more common human parasites as the use of broad-spectrum pesticides for other insect pests has declined.

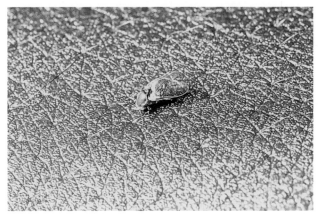

Fig. 4.113. *Simulium*, the black fly or buffalo gnat, has worldwide distribution. These small flies have a humpbacked appearance. Eggs are laid in rapidly flowing water. In large numbers, black flies cause irritation, dermatitis, and even fatal toxemia or exsanguination. Photo courtesy of Dr. Jeffrey F. Williams, Vanson HaloSource, Inc., Redmond, WA.

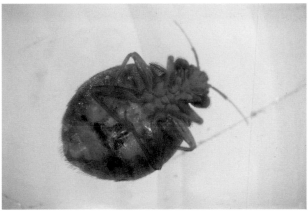

Fig. 4.114. Adult bedbug, *Cimex* sp., from a motel in Florida, USA.

Parasites of Fish

Stephen A. Smith, Virginia-Maryland
Regional College of Veterinary Medicine,
Virginia Tech, Blacksburg, VA

Fish can serve as definitive, intermediate, or paratenic (transport) hosts in the life cycle of many species of protozoan, metazoan, and crustacean parasites. Most of these parasites can be readily identified microscopically, and as with mammalian parasites, the correct identification and an understanding of their life cycle are important in the prevention or management of an outbreak of disease due to parasites.

Protozoan parasites probably cause more disease in both ornamental and cultured fish than any other group of parasites. An example of a common parasitic disease is white spot disease, or "ich," caused by *Ichthyophthirius multifiliis* in freshwater fish and by *Cryptocaryon irritans* in marine species.

Metazoan parasites can be found as larval or adult forms in almost every tissue of fish. Most can be grossly identified as monogeneans, digenetic trematodes, nematodes, cestodes, acanthocephalans, or crustaceans, but specific identification generally involves special staining techniques or clearing of specimens.

Examples of common fish helminths include monogeneans on the gills and skin; larval digenetic trematodes (metacercariae) in the eyes, skin, musculature, and abdominal cavity; larval cestodes and nematodes in the visceral organs and abdominal cavity; and an assortment of adult trematodes, nematodes, cestodes, and acanthocephalans in the lumen of the gastrointestinal tract. In addition, a number of arthropod parasites and leeches can be found occurring on or attached to the skin and fins.

TECHNIQUES FOR RECOVERY OF ECTOPARASITES

A variety of nonlethal techniques that include skin, fin, and gill biopsies have been developed for the diagnosis of the common external parasites of fish. Most of these biopsy techniques can be performed on live fish without the use of anesthesia, although light sedation often simplifies the procedure and makes it less stressful for the fish.

Skin Biopsy (Mucus Smear)

The skin is the primary target organ for many of the external fish parasites. Therefore, a biopsy of the skin (Fig. 5.1) is one of the most useful and common samples for diagnosing ectoparasitic problems. This biopsy is performed by gently scraping a small area on the surface of the fish with a scalpel blade or the edge of a microscope coverslip in a cranial to caudal direction. Care should be taken to use only a minimal amount of pressure to obtain this superficial scraping, since deeper damage to the skin may result in secondary bacterial infections or osmoregulatory imbalance in the fish.

The mucus from the skin scraping should be transferred immediately to a drop of aquarium water (either fresh or salt water depending on the species of fish, but *not* city tap water) on a glass microscope slide and a coverslip carefully applied. This wet mount should then be examined under the compound microscope for the presence of free-swimming, attached, or encysted protozoan or metazoan parasites.

Fin Biopsy (Fin "Snip")

A fin biopsy (Fig. 5.2) is obtained by snipping a small piece of tissue from the peripheral edge of one of the fins. This procedure is often less traumatic to the fish than a skin biopsy, since a smaller wound is generally produced. The fin snip should be transferred immediately to a drop of aquarium or pond water on a glass microscope slide, spread to its full extent, and a coverslip carefully applied. This wet mount should then be examined under the microscope for the presence of protozoan or metazoan parasites.

Gill Biopsy (Gill "Snip")

A gill biopsy (Fig. 5.3) is obtained by inserting the tip of a pair of fine scissors into the branchial cavity behind the operculum (gill cover) and cutting off the distal ends of several of the primary gill lamellae attached to the gill arch. Since only the tips of the primary lamellae are removed, minimal bleeding should occur. The gill tissue should be transferred immediately to a drop of aquarium or pond water on a glass microscope slide, the individual lamellae separated, and a coverslip carefully applied. This wet mount should then be examined under the microscope for the presence of protozoan or metazoan parasites.

RECOVERY OF ENDOPARASITES

Examination of fish feces for the presence of internal parasites is accomplished with the same techniques as those used for mammals and birds. A fresh fecal sample is collected with a pipette either from the bottom of the aquarium or as it hangs from the vent of the fish. If an appropriate sample cannot be acquired from the environment or if examination of a specific individual is desired, the application of gentle pressure on the sides of a netted fish often produces the desired sample. The fecal specimen is then processed by standard flotation or sedimentation techniques and evaluated for the presence of parasite eggs and larvae. Though specific parasite identification is generally impossible, fecal examination does provide useful information about the types of parasites (nematodes, trematodes, cestodes, acanthocephalans) that may be present in a fish.

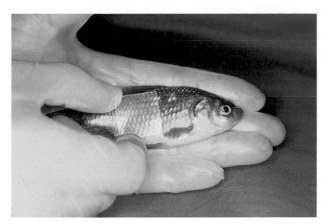

Fig. 5.1. Collection of mucus sample via a skin biopsy from the side of a fish for external-parasite examination.

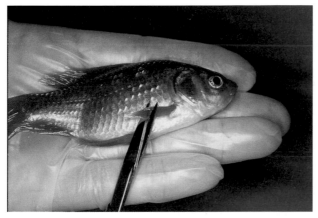

Fig. 5.2. Collection of a fin biopsy by clipping a small portion of the distal tip of the pectoral fin.

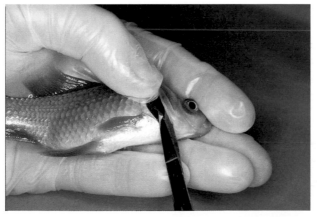

Fig. 5.3. Collection of a gill biopsy by lifting the operculum (gill chamber cover) and removing a few distal filaments (lamellae) of the gill.

PARASITES OF FISH

PARASITE: *Ichthyophthirius multifiliis* (Figures 5.4–5.5)
Common name: "Ich" or freshwater white spot disease.

Taxonomy: Protozoan (ciliate).

Geographic Distribution: Freshwater fish worldwide.

Location in Host: Beneath the surface epithelial layer of skin, fins, and gills.

Life Cycle: These parasites have a direct life cycle, with free-swimming, ciliated tomites (theronts) in water invading the skin, fins, and gills of fish. The tomites penetrate deep into the epithelial tissues and form large, feeding trophozoites (trophonts) that eventually excyst from the host and enter the water, where each develops into a cyst. The cyst stage then undergoes multiple divisions, producing numerous infectious tomites that are released to the environment to infect other fish hosts.

Laboratory Diagnosis: This large, holotrich ciliate with a characteristic C-shaped nucleus is detected in wet mounts of skin biopsies and gill and fin snips.

Size:	trophozoites	up to 1 mm in diameter
	tomites in water column	25–50 μm × 15–22 μm

Clinical Importance: The parasite causes small, raised, white lesions on skin, fins, and gill tissue. Penetration into and excystation out of the epithelial tissue by the parasite cause loss of integrity of external tissues and result in disruption of normal homeostatic osmoregulatory processes.

PARASITE: *Cryptocaryon irritans* (Figure 5.5)
Common name: Marine white spot disease.

Taxonomy: Protozoan (ciliate).

Geographic Distribution: Marine and brackish water fish worldwide.

Location in Host: Beneath the surface epithelial layer of skin, fins, and gills.

Life Cycle: The life cycle is the same as that of the freshwater *Ichthyophthirius multifiliis:* free-swimming ciliated tomites in water invade the skin, fins, and gills, penetrate deep into the epithelial tissues, and form large, feeding trophozoites that eventually excyst from the host into the water and develop into cysts. The cyst stage then undergoes multiple divisions, producing numerous infectious tomites that are released to the environment to infect other fish hosts.

Laboratory Diagnosis: This holotrich ciliate, which does *not* have a C-shaped nucleus, is detected in wet mounts of skin biopsies and gill and fin snips.

Size:	trophozoites	up to 1 mm in diameter
	tomites in water	25–50 μm × 15–22 μm

Clinical Importance: *Cryptocaryon* causes small, raised, white lesions on skin, fins, and gill tissue. Penetration into and excystation out of host epithelial tissue by the parasite cause loss of integrity of external tissues and result in disruption of normal homeostatic osmoregulatory processes.

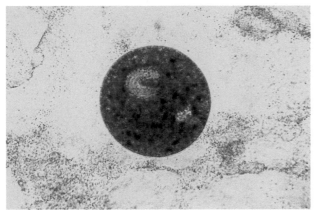

Fig. 5.4. *Ichthyophthirius multifiliis* trophozoite. This ciliate, which appears as small, raised, white bumps on the skin, fins, and gills of fish, is commonly called "ich" or white spot disease. This parasite varies in size, ranging from 100 to 1000 μm, depending on the stage of maturation, available nutrition, and host species.

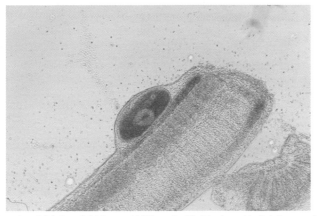

Fig. 5.5. Encysted trophozoite of *Ichthyophthirius multifiliis* embedded in the epithelial tissues of a gill filament of a goldfish. *Cryptocaryon irritans* is a similar organism in marine fish species.

Parasite: *Tetrahymena* **spp.** (Figure 5.6)

Taxonomy: Protozoan (ciliate). Species include *T. corlissi* and *T. pyriformis.*

Geographic Distribution: Freshwater fish and amphibians worldwide.

Location in Host: Trophozoites are generally found on surface epithelial layers of skin and fins but may be found in deeper skin tissues, muscle, and abdominal organs.

Life Cycle: In the freshwater environment this parasite forms reproductive cysts in which 2–8 infectious tomites are produced.

Laboratory Diagnosis: Small, cylindrical- to pyriform-shaped ciliates are found in wet mounts of skin biopsies.

    Size: trophozoite   55 μm × 30 μm

Clinical Importance: This facultative parasite is histophagous and invades the skin, muscle, and internal organs, causing osmoregulatory and body system dysfunction.

Parasite: *Uronema* **spp.,** including *U. marinum* (Figure 5.7)

Taxonomy: Protozoan (ciliate).

Geographic Distribution: Marine fish worldwide.

Location in Host: Surface epithelial layers of skin and fins of marine fish but also in deeper skin tissues, muscle, and abdominal organs.

Life Cycle: This parasite (similar to freshwater *Tetrahymena* spp.) forms reproductive cysts in the marine environment in which several infectious tomites are produced.

Laboratory Diagnosis: Small, cylindrical- to pyriform-shaped ciliates are found in wet mounts of skin biopsies.

    Size: trophozoite   50 μm × 30 μm

Clinical Importance: This facultative, histophagous parasite (similar to freshwater *Tetrahymena* spp.) invades the skin, muscle, and internal organs, causing osmoregulatory and body system dysfunction.

Parasite: *Epistylis* **spp.** (Figure 5.8)

Taxonomy: Protozoan (ciliate). Species include *E. colisarum* and *E. lwoffi.*

Geographic Distribution: Freshwater fish worldwide.

Location in Host: Attached to surface epithelial layers of skin and fins.

Life Cycle: This parasite divides by binary fission along the longitudinal axis, producing two daughter cells.

Laboratory Diagnosis: This colonial ciliate is detected in wet mounts of the skin and is identified by its conical or elongated cylindrical body, a noncontractile stalk, and a thin, epistomal disk for attachment.

    Size: 150–300 μm × 40–60 μm

Clinical Importance: The epistomal disk causes a localized skin lesion and mechanical disruption of the normal osmoregulatory process of the skin. Generally, fish develop skin lesions only in heavy infestations.

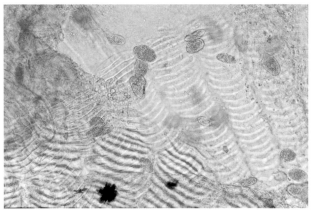

Fig. 5.6. Numerous trophozoites of *Tetrahymena* spp. in a skin biopsy of a hybrid striped bass. This small ciliate also infects many species of ornamental aquarium fish.

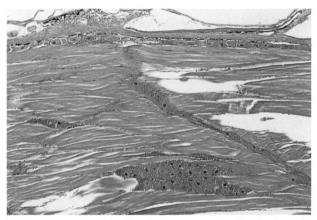

Fig. 5.7. Tissue section showing numerous trophozoites of *Uronema* spp. invading the deeper tissues of a marine flounder species. This organism causes pathology similar to that of *Tetrahymena* spp. of freshwater species of fish.

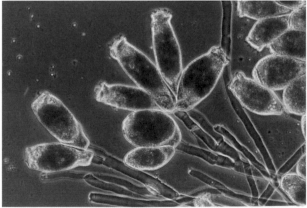

Fig. 5.8. *Epistylis* sp. is a colonial ciliate that has a conical or elongated cylindrical body, a noncontractile stalk, and an epistomal disk for attachment to the host. The parasite generally causes localized skin lesions only in heavy infestations.

PARASITE: *Trichodina* **spp.** (Figure 5.9)

Taxonomy: Protozoan (ciliate). Related species include *Trichodinella* spp., *Hemitrichodina* spp., *Dipartiella* spp., *Paratrichodina* spp., and *Tripartiella* spp.

Geographic Distribution: Freshwater, brackish, and marine fish worldwide.

Location in Host: Surface layers of skin, fins, and gills.

Life Cycle: This parasite divides by binary fission, producing two daughter cells.

Laboratory Diagnosis: This flattened, circular, ciliated protozoan is detected in wet mounts of skin biopsies and gill and fin snips and is identified by its prominent denticular (toothlike) internal ring and its ventrally located concave adhesive disk.

Size: variable, 150–300 μm × 40–60 μm

Clinical Importance: These organisms are usually ectocommensal but become ectoparasitic when environmental and host conditions are suitable. This scrub-brush-like parasite may cause localized to generalized skin lesions and disruption of the normal respiratory process of the gill and osmoregulatory process of the skin. Generally, it is only a problem in heavy infestations of the skin and gill, though a few species are parasitic inhabitants of the urinary tract of fish.

PARASITE: *Trichophyra* **sp.** (Figure 5.10)

Taxonomy: Protozoan (ciliate).

Geographic Distribution: Freshwater fish worldwide.

Location in Host: Attached to epithelial surfaces of the skin, fins, and gills.

Life Cycle: This parasite reproduces by endogenous budding.

Laboratory Diagnosis: This small, sedentary organism with suctorial tentacles can usually be observed in wet mounts of gill snips.

Size: 30–50 μm

Clinical Importance: This parasite is generally only a problem in heavy infestations, where this pincushion-like ciliate attaches to the skin, fin, and gill tissues and causes irritation and localized lesions that disrupt normal respiratory and osmoregulatory processes of the fish.

PARASITE: *Amyloodinium ocellatum* (Figures 5.11–5.12)
         Common name: Velvet disease or rust disease.

Taxonomy: Protozoan (flagellate).

Geographic Distribution: Marine fish worldwide.

Location in Host: Attached to epithelial tissues of skin, fins, and gills.

Life Cycle: The trophozoite attaches to the host via an attachment disk with filiform projections that embed into the epithelial tissue of the host. The trophozoite detaches from the host and forms an encysted tomont that divides and produces up to 256 free-swimming, infective dinospores.

Laboratory Diagnosis: Large, cylindrical dinoflagellates may be seen in wet mounts of gill snips where the organism is attached to filaments of the gill tissue.

Size: up to 150–200 μm in length

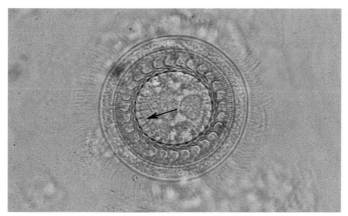

Fig. 5.9. *Trichodina* sp. from a skin biopsy of an aquarium Oscar. These flattened ciliates have a prominent circular, denticular ring (*arrow*), upon which specific identification is based.

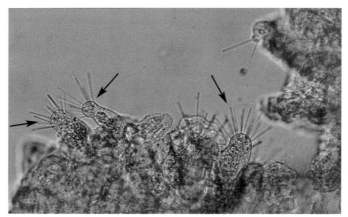

Fig. 5.10. *Trichophyra* sp. on a gill biopsy of a channel catfish. This freshwater protozoan parasite has a "pincushion" appearance (*arrows*) and is often found on the skin and gills of pond-reared fish.

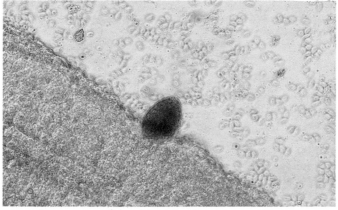

Fig. 5.11. *Amyloodinium ocellatum* on the gill tissue of a striped bass. This organism is the cause of "velvet" or "rust" in marine species of fish. *Oodinium* sp. is a similar organism in freshwater fish.

273

Clinical Importance: This ectoparasite causes irritation of the gill, resulting in hyperplasia of the epithelial tissues and fusion of gill lamellae. Outbreaks may be fatal in heavily infected fish, especially in fish that are weakened or stressed by other conditions.

PARASITE: *Ichthyobodo* (= *Costia*) *necator* (Figure 5.13)

Taxonomy: Protozoan (flagellate).

Geographic Distribution: Freshwater fish worldwide.

Location in Host: Attached to epithelial tissues of skin, fins, and gills.

Life Cycle: The attached, feeding stage alternates with a free-swimming nonfeeding stage.

Laboratory Diagnosis: This very small flagellate with two unequal flagella extending from its posteriolateral groove is detected in wet mounts of skin biopsies and gill snips.

Size: 5 μm × 10 μm

Clinical Importance: This often overlooked parasite is extremely pathogenic in young fish and older fish with lowered resistance. *Icthyobodo* causes irritation of the skin and gill tissue, resulting in hyperplasia of the epithelial tissues and fusion of gill lamellae.

PARASITE: *Henneguya* spp. (Figure 5.14)

Taxonomy: Protozoan (myxospora). Many genera and species.

Geographic Distribution: Freshwater and marine fish worldwide.

Location in Host: Gills and skin but may also invade internal organs.

Life Cycle: Plasmodia develop within polysporic cysts in the epithelial cells of the gill or skin.

Laboratory Diagnosis: Variable-sized cysts found within wet mounts of gill tissue contain spores with ellipsoidal, rounded, or spindle-shaped smooth valves.

Size: 19 μm × 4.5 μm, with two caudal appendages of 45 μm each

Clinical Importance: Parasite development causes a hyperplastic reaction in epithelial cells of the gills, causing severe branchitis with respiratory compromise. This protozoan is a significant pathogen of the commercial catfish industry.

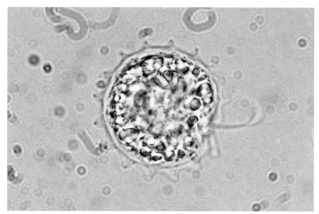

Fig. 5.12. Free-swimming dinospore stage of *Amyloodinium ocellatum,* which is infectious to many species of marine fish.

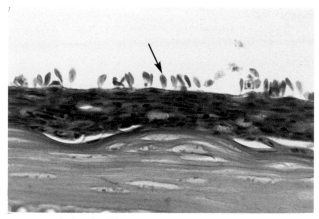

Fig. 5.13. *Ichthyobodo necator*, attached to the skin (*arrow*), is an extremely pathogenic species of flagellate of freshwater fish that is often overlooked due to its small size.

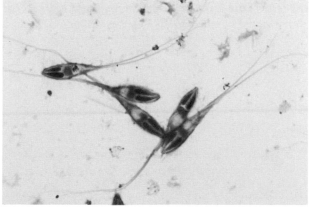

Fig. 5.14. Giemsa-stained spores of *Henneguya* sp. (a myxosporidian) from a ruptured cyst in the gill filament of a freshwater channel catfish. Note the two anterior polar capsules within the spore and forked caudal appendages.

PARASITE: Monogenetic Flukes (Figure 5.15)

Taxonomy: Trematodes (Monogenea).

Geographic Distribution: Freshwater and marine fish worldwide.

Location in Host: Attached to skin, fins, and gills.

Life Cycle: Monogeneans complete their viviparous or ovoviviparous life cycle on one host. Eggs often have polar elongations. Larvae are often morphologically similar to adults.

Laboratory Diagnosis: These small- to medium-sized flatworms have a posterior attachment organ, or haptor, that may have hooks, anchors, clamps, or suckers. Monogeneans are commonly found in wet mounts of gill snips or skin biopsies.

Size: up to 5 mm

Clinical Importance: These parasitic flatworms cause damage at the site of attachment and also through their feeding activity on the surface of the host fish.

PARASITE: Larval Flukes (Figure 5.16)

Taxonomy: Trematodes (Digenea).

Geographic Distribution: Freshwater and marine fish worldwide.

Location in Host: Encysted metacercariae can be found in any tissue of the fish, including the skin, muscle, eyes, brain, and visceral organs.

Life Cycle: Digenetic trematodes require at least one intermediate host, commonly a snail or other mollusk, to complete their life cycle. Eggs are deposited in water by the carnivorous definitive host (mammal, bird, or fish), hatch, and release free-swimming miracidia that enter a first intermediate snail host. Parasites emerge from the snail as free-swimming cercariae that penetrate the tissue of the second intermediate fish host. The parasites then become either encysted or unencysted metacercariae. They do not complete their development until ingested by an appropriate carnivorous host (e.g., fish-eating birds, fish, or mammals).

Laboratory Diagnosis: Immature trematodes are generally grossly visible within a cyst.

Size: Variable, up to several millimeters

Clinical Importance: These parasites may be unsightly in tissues but generally are of minimal significance unless large numbers of metacercariae interfere with organ function.

PARASITE: *Argulus* spp. (Figure 5.17)

Taxonomy: Arthropod (crustacean).

Geographic Distribution: Freshwater and marine fish worldwide.

Location in Host: Generally on the skin and fins.

Life Cycle: Eggs, laid in water, release free-swimming copepod larvae that attach to suitable fish hosts and metamorphose several to numerous times before reaching the adult stage.

Laboratory Diagnosis: This grossly visible dorsoventrally flattened, oval parasite has two prominent sucking disks, two dark-colored eyespots, and a centrally located piercing stylet.

Size: 3–5 mm

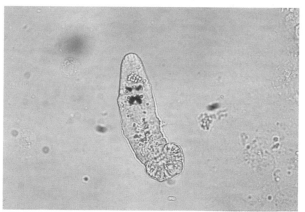

Fig. 5.15. Adult monogenean collected from the skin of a rainbow trout. These external parasites have hooks, anchors, clamps, or suckers for attachment to the skin, fins, and gills.

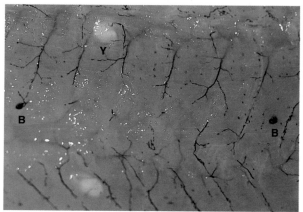

Fig. 5.16. Encysted metacercariae of two different species of digenetic trematodes in the muscle of a bluegill. The smaller organism (B) is commonly called "black spot disease" (*Neascus* sp.), and the larger, paler one (Y) is commonly called a "yellow grub" (*Clinostomum* sp.). Both are larval stages that will not complete metamorphosis until ingested by a carnivorous host.

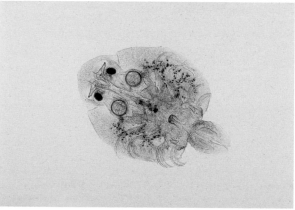

Fig. 5.17. *Argulus* from a goldfish, commonly known as a "fish louse." This ectoparasitic crustacean can be found on the skin and fins of freshwater fish. Other species can be found on brackish and marine species of fish.

Clinical Importance: This crustacean causes damage by piercing the host and sucking blood, often resulting in a severe localized reaction at the site of stylet penetration. These parasitic arthropods may be important vectors in the transmission of certain viral, bacterial, and protozoal fish diseases.

PARASITE: Leeches (Figure 5.18)

Taxonomy: Phylum Annelida, class Hirudinea.

Geographic Distribution: Freshwater and marine fish worldwide.

Location in Host: Attached to skin, fins, and gills.

Life Cycle: Leeches periodically attach to fish to ingest a blood meal.

Laboratory Diagnosis: These grossly visible flat to cylindrical wormlike organisms have a varying number of divisions and generally both anterior and posterior suckers.

Size: variable, up to several centimeters in length

Clinical Importance: Besides the physical damage caused by attachment and bloodsucking activities, leeches are vectors for a variety of fish pathogens, including viruses, bacteria, and blood parasites.

PARASITE: Thorny-Headed Worms of Fish (Figure 5.19)

Taxonomy: Phylum Acanthocephala.

Geographic Distribution: Freshwater and marine fish worldwide.

Location in Host: Lumen of posterior intestinal tract.

Life Cycle: These parasites have an indirect life cycle, with usually a crustacean intermediate host.

Laboratory Diagnosis: Eggs are observed on standard fecal flotation or direct smear.

Size: 50–65 × 30–40 μm

Clinical Importance: These parasites generally do not cause any clinical signs in fish. Rarely, a severe infection will result from perforation of the intestinal tract, with subsequent peritonitis.

PARASITE: Nematode Parasites (Figure 5.20)

Taxonomy: Nematodes belonging to various orders.

Geographic Distribution: Freshwater and marine fish worldwide.

Location in Host: Lumen of intestinal tract.

Life Cycle: A variety of direct and indirect life cycles have been reported.

Laboratory Diagnosis: A variety of nematode-type eggs may be observed on standard fecal flotation or direct smear.

Size: variable

Clinical Importance: Adult nematode parasites generally do not cause any clinical signs in fish. A severe infection sometimes will result in mechanical blockage of the intestinal tract and/or chronic weight loss.

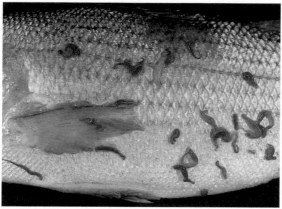

Fig. 5.18. Leeches of an unidentified species on the skin of a cultured hybrid striped bass.

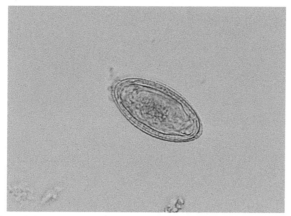

Fig. 5.19. Egg of an acanthocephalan parasite from a black crappie.

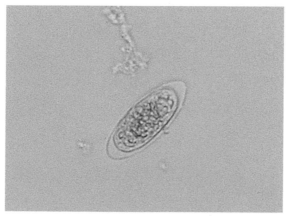

Fig. 5.20. Unidentified nematode egg from a largemouth bass.

Selected and
Cited References

Barnard S. M., and Upton S. J. 1996. A Veterinary Guide to the Parasites of Reptiles: Protozoa. Krieger Publishing Co., Malabar, FL.

BonDurant, R. H. 1985. Diagnosis, treatment, and control of bovine trichomoniasis. Comp. Cont. Ed. Vet. Prac. 7:S179–S188.

Bowman, D. D. 2003. Georgis' Parasitology for Veterinarians. 8th ed. Saunders, St. Louis, MO.

Bowman, D. D., Hendrix, C. M., Lindsay, D. S., and Barr, S. C. 2002. Feline Clinical Parasitology. Iowa State University Press, Ames.

Clyde, V. L., and Patton S. 1996. Diagnosis, treatment and control of common parasites in companion and avian birds. Seminars in Avian and Exotic Pet Medicine 5:75–84.

Coles, G. C., Bauer, C., Borgsteede, F. H. M., Geerts, S., Klei, T. R., Taylor, M. A., and Waller, P. J. 1992. World Association for the Advancement of Veterinary Parasitology (W.A.A.V.P.) methods for the detection of anthelmintic resistance in nematodes of veterinary importance. Vet. Parasitol. 44:35–44.

Feldman, B. V., Zinkl, J. G., and Jain, N. C. 2000. Schalm's Veterinary Hematology. Lippincott Williams & Wilkins, Philadelphia.

Flynn, R.J. 1973. Parasites of Laboratory Animals. Iowa State University Press, Ames.

Foreyt, W. J. 1997. Veterinary Parasitology Reference Manual. Iowa State University Press, Ames.

Fowler, M. F. 1998. Parasites. In Medicine and Surgery of South American Camelids, 2nd ed., by M. F. Fowler, 195–230. Iowa State University Press.

Garcia, L. S. 2001. Diagnostic Medical Parasitology. ASM Press, Washington, DC.

Georgi, J. R., and Georgi M. E. 1992. Canine Clinical Parasitology. Lea & Febiger, Philadelphia.

Gookin, J. L., Foster, D. M., Poore, M. F., Stebbins, M. E., and Levy, M. G. 2003. Use of a commercially available culture system for diagnosis of *Tritrichomonas foetus* infection in cats. J. Am. Vet. Med. Assoc. 222:1376–1379.

Gratzek, J. B. 1988. Parasites associated with ornamental fish. In Veterinary Clinics of North America: Small Animal Practice, ed. M. K. Stoskopf, 18:375–400.

Greiner, E. C., and Ritchie B. W. 1994. Parasites. In Avian Medicine: Principles and Application, ed. B. W. Ritchie, G. J. Harrison, and L. R. Harrison, 1007–1029. Wingers Publishing Co., Lake Worth, FL.

Hendricks, C. M. 2002. Laboratory Procedures for Veterinary Technicians. 4th ed. Mosby, St. Louis, MO.

Hoffman, G. L. 1999. Parasites of North American Freshwater Fishes. Cornell University Press, Ithaca.

Jacobs, D. E. 1986. A Colour Atlas of Equine Parasites. Gower Medical Publishing, London.

Kassai, T. 1999. Veterinary Helminthology. Butterworth-Heinemann Publishing, Oxford.

Kaufmann, J. 1996. Parasitic Infections of Domestic Animals. Birkhäuser Verlag, Boston.

Kennedy, M.J., Mackinnon, J. D., and Higgs, G. W. 1998. Veterinary Parasitology: Laboratory Procedures. Alberta Agriculture, Food and Rural Development Publishing Branch, Edmonton.

Kettle, D. S. 1995. Medical and Veterinary Entomology. 2nd ed. CAB International, Wallingford, UK.

Levine, N. D. 1980. Nematode Parasites of Domestic Animals and Man. 2nd ed. Burgess Publishing, Minneapolis.

Lom, J., and Dykova, I. 1992. Protozoan Parasites of Fishes. Developments in Aquaculture and Fisheries Science 26. Elsevier, Amsterdam.

Ministry of Agriculture, Fisheries and Food. 1986. Manual of Veterinary Parasitological Laboratory Techniques. Reference Book 418. Her Majesty's Stationery Office, London.

Mullen, G., and Durden, L. 2003. Medical and Veterinary Entomology. Academic Press, New York.

Neimester, R., Logan, A. L., Gerber, B., Egleton, J. H., and Kleger, B. 1987. Hemo-De as a substitute for ethyl acetate in formalin-ethyl acetate concentration technique. J. Clin. Microbiol. 25:425–426.

Owen, D. G. 1992. Parasites of Laboratory Animals. Royal Society of Medicine Services, London.

Roberts, R. J. 2001. The parasitology of teleosts. In Fish Pathology, 3rd ed., ed. R. J. Roberts, 254–296. W. B. Saunders, Philadelphia.

Smith, S. A. 1996. Parasites of birds of prey: Their diagnosis and treatment. Seminars in Avian and Exotic Pet Medicine 5:97–105.

——. 2002. Non-lethal clinical techniques used in the diagnosis of fish diseases. Journal of the American Veterinary Medicine Association 220:1203–1206.

Smith, S. A., and Noga, E. J. 1992. General parasitology of fish. In Fish Medicine, ed. M. K. Stoskopf, 131–148. W. B. Saunders, Philadelphia.

Soulsby, E. J. L. 1965. Textbook of Veterinary Clinical Parasitology. F. A. Davis Co., Philadelphia.

——. 1982. Helminths, Arthropods, and Protozoa of Domesticated Animals. 7th ed. Williams & Wilkins, Baltimore.

Taira, N., Ando, Y., and Williams, J. C. 2003. A Color Atlas of Clinical Helminthology of Domestic Animals. Elsevier Science, Amsterdam.

Thienpont, D., Rochette, F., and Vanparijs, O. F. J. 1979. Diagnosing Helminthiasis through Coprological Examination. Janssen Research Foundation, Beerse, Belgium.

Urquhart, G. M., Armour, J., Duncan, J. L., Dunn, A. M., and Jennings, F. W. 1996. Veterinary Parasitology. 2nd ed. Blackwell Science, London.

U.S. Department of Agriculture. 1976. Ticks of Veterinary Importance. Agriculture Handbook 485. U.S. Government Printing Office, Washington, DC.

Wall, R., and Shearer, D. 2001. Veterinary Ectoparasites: Biology, Pathology and Control. Blackwell Science, London.

Willams, J. F. W., and Zajac, A. 1980. Diagnosis of Gastrointestinal Parasites in Dogs and Cats. Ralston Purina, St. Louis, MO.

Williams, R. E., Hall, R. D., Broce, A. B., and Scholl, P. J. 1985. Livestock Entomology. John Wiley & Sons, New York.

Wison, S. C., and Carpenter, J. W. 1996. Endoparasitic disease of reptiles. Seminars in Avian and Exotic Pet Medicine 5:64–74.

Zajac, A. M., Johnson, J., and King, S. E. 2002. Evaluation of the importance of centrifugation as a component of zinc sulfate fecal flotation examinations. J. Am. Anim. Hosp. Assoc. 38:221–224.

Index

Page references given in *italics* refer to illustrations.